30 Day Whole Diet

The Essential Whole Foods Cookbook for Beginners

Trustworthy Recipes for Weight Loss and Healthy Living

Emma Green

Copyright © 2018 by Emma Green.

All rights reserved.

No part of this book may be reproduced in any form or by any electronic or mechanical means – except in the case of brief quotation embodied in articles or reviews – without written permission from its publisher.

Disclaimer

The recipes and information in this book are provided for educational purposes only. Please always consult a licensed professional before making changes to your lifestyle or diet. The author and/or publisher shall have neither liability nor responsibility to anyone with respect to any loss or damage caused or alleged to be caused directly or indirectly by the information contained in this book. All trademarks and brands within this book are for clarifying purposes only and are owned by the owners themselves, not affiliated with this document.

Images from shutterstock.com

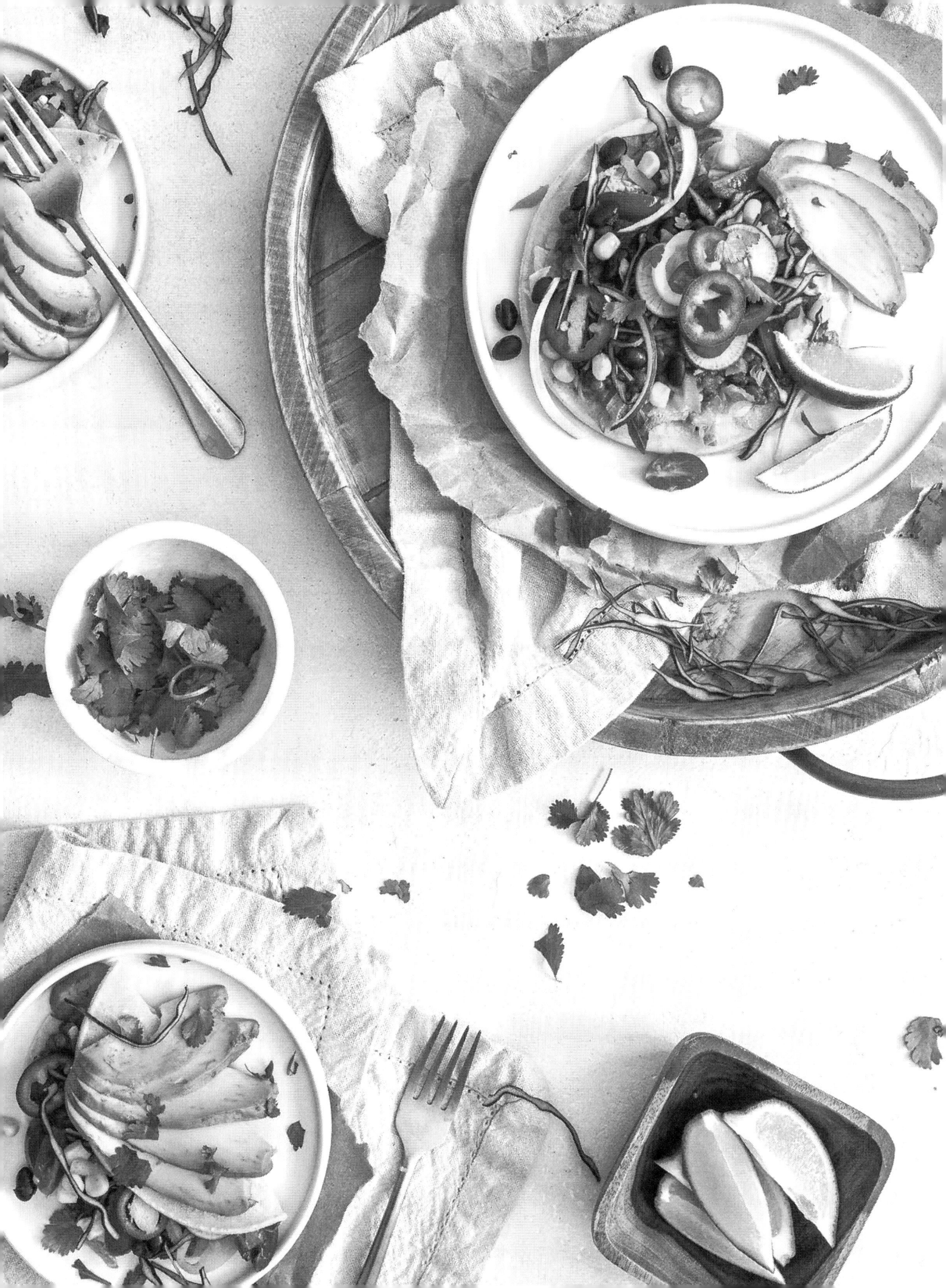

CONTENTS

INTRODUCTION 6

Chapter 1. The Basics 7
- What is Whole Food? 7
- 7 Good Reasons to Eat Whole Foods 7
- What are the 30 Days of Whole Food? 9
- Foods to Eat 11
- Foods to Avoid 13
- Tips for the Whole Food Diet 14
- The Essential Five 16
- Setting Up a Whole Food Kitchen and Pantry 18

Chapter 2. Recipes 19

BREAKFAST 19
- Oatmeal Fruit Shake 19
- Pumpkin Pie Smoothie 20
- Breakfast Green Machine Smoothie 21
- Breakfast Sandwich 22
- Veggie and Tofu Scramble 23
- Breakfast Banana Splits 24
- Whole Wheat Blueberry Pancakes 25
- Kasha Breakfast Porridge 26
- Breakfast Turkey Sausage 27
- Mini Sausage Breakfast Sandwiches 28
- Amaranth Banana Breakfast Porridge 29
- Orangeade 30

LUNCH 31
- Deviled Ham Tea Sandwiches 31
- Oil-Free Herb Pesto 32
- Refried Bean and Avocado Soft Tacos 33
- Fresh Salsa 34
- Veggies, Herbs Salad, and Orange-Miso Tahini Dressing 35

SOUPS & SALADS 36
- Spicy Squash Soup 36
- Spicy Tortilla Soup with Black Beans 37
- Salmon Chowder 38
- Summer Borscht 39
- King Oyster Mushroom Soup 40
- Black Bean Salad with Avocado-Lime Dressing 41
- Tangy Bean Salad with Carrots and Green Onions 42
- Seafood Salad 43
- Quinoa, Chard, and Apple Salad 44
- Salade Niçoise 45

 Arugula Salad with Butternut Squash and Prosciutto 46

BOWLS 47

 Mighty Bowl of Goodness 47
 Red Pepper Pico 48
 Avocado-Jalapeño Crème 49
 Buddha Bowl 50

DINNER 51

 Mock Chicken Nuggets 51
 Grilled Chicken and Vegetable Dinner 52
 Tarragon Roasted Chicken 53
 Beef Tacos 54
 Mini Turkey Meatloaf and Green Beans Dinner 55
 Bacon-Wrapped Stuffed Sea Scallops 56
 Grilled Chicken and Peppers over Arugula 57
 Grilled Caribbean Pork Tenderloin 58
 Roasted Lemon-Herb Chicken 59
 Pesto Chicken Breasts 60
 Lemon-Thyme Roasted Capon 61
 Mustard Grilled Lamb Chops 62
 Herb-Rubbed Bison Steaks 63
 Pear-Sage Meatloaf 64
 Venison Burgers 65

DESSERTS 66

 Sweet Potato Chocolate Mousse 66
 Raspberry Nice Cream 67
 Coconut Cookies 68
 Fruit and Waffle Kabobs 69
 Oatmeal-Raisin Cookies 70
 Star Anise Pears 71

CONCLUSION 72

Recipe Index 73

Conversion Tables 74

Other Books by Emma Green 75

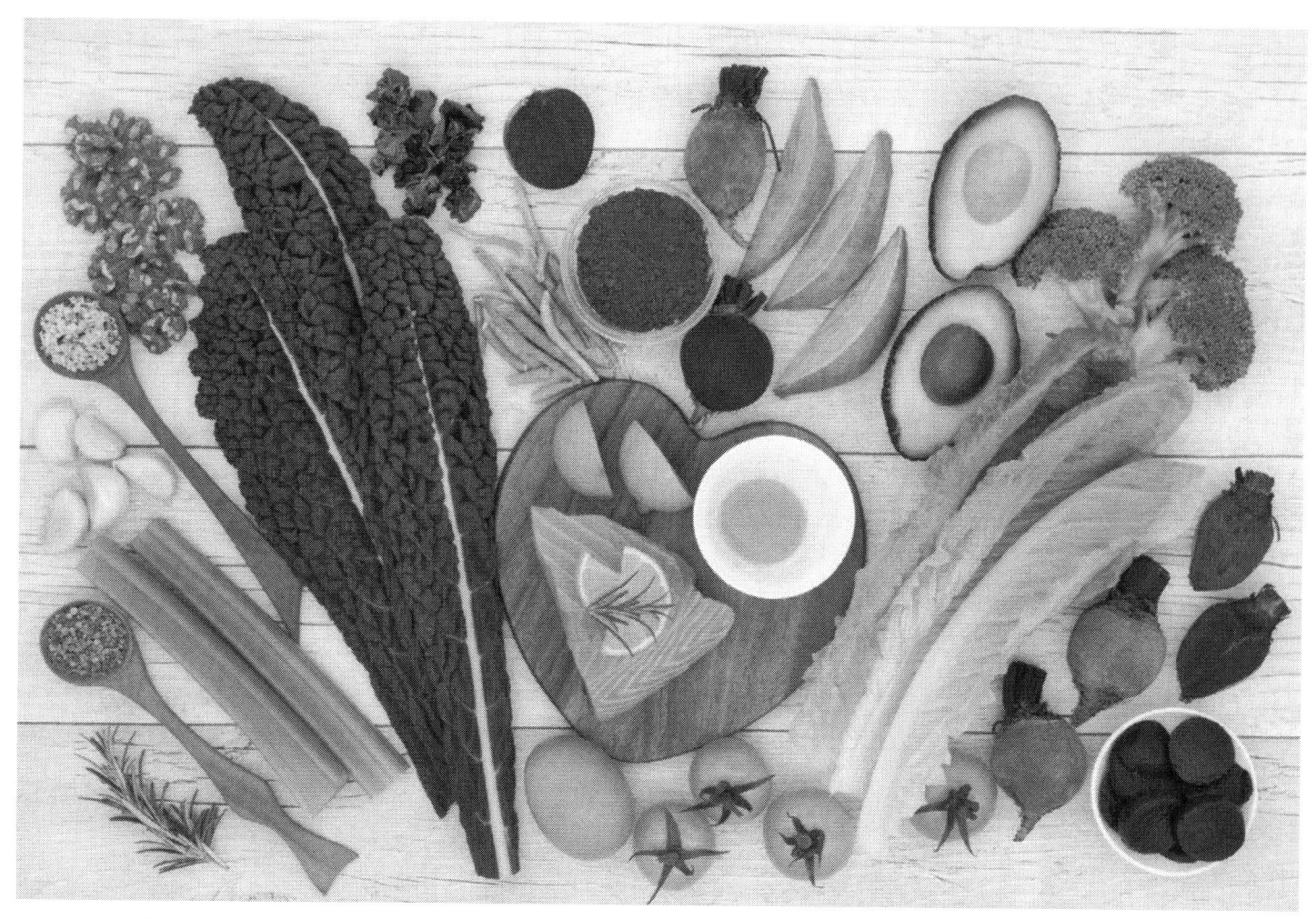

INTRODUCTION

Diet and environment have changed dramatically over the last years. With these changes have come rising rates of obesity, skin disorders, cancer, heart disease, diabetes, and more.

More and more studies advise us to eat how our ancestors used to eat hundreds of years ago. Recent research made by nutritionists has pointed in the direction of eating whole foods, or foods that are as close to their natural form as they possibly can be. Consuming more whole foods is better for improving your health and preventing diseases. Fruits, vegetables, nuts, whole grains, and legumes contain thousands of important phytochemicals that work with our bodies to build and maintain optimal health. Eating food is so much more than a way to fill our bellies. Food affects our quality of life, how we look, how we feel, how much we weigh, how much energy we have, how we age, and how healthy we are.

The book you are holding gives proven steps and strategies on how to eat nothing but whole foods for 30 days. It was written for anyone who wants to change their lives for the better, starting with a healthy and beneficial diet. Give yourself 30 days to make that change, and you will never regret it. You deserve to have a healthy and fit body. There is no better time to start than now!

Chapter 1. The Basics

What is Whole Food?

Whole foods are considered the foods that are very close to their whole and natural state. They can be, for example, fresh vegetables and fruits, nuts and seeds, whole grains, dried beans, and fresh wild salmon. Whole foods have not been processed in any way that would disturb their nutrition or flavor. They don`t contain flavorings, solvents, chemical preservatives, food dyes, and many others.

Whole foods have not had any parts removed from them. These foods retain all of the nutrients to properly digest and metabolize themselves. For example, white rice is only part of brown rice (the nutrient-rich germ and bran parts have been removed), and cornstarch is only part of the whole corn kernel.

By eating whole foods, you keep things out of your body that can contribute to many health problems. For example, the flavor enhancer MSG is found in many foods, including processed "health foods," like yeast extract, calcium caseinate, and hydrolyzed vegetable protein. It may be a little bit hard to have every part of your diet be a whole food. Some foods that are still close to their whole forms, such as extra-virgin olive oil and natural sweeteners, can be used without compromising your health.

7 Good Reasons to Eat Whole Foods

1. **Promote Intestinal Function**

You may not believe it, but there are more microorganisms in the human intestinal tract than there are stars in the universe. Some bacteria help us to manufacture vitamins, digest our food and amino acids, repair our intestinal cells, and even calm our immune systems. Foods such as raw cultured vegetables, raw sauerkraut, unpasteurized miso, and kombucha are sources of these beneficial bacteria. Many plant foods, such as apricots, asparagus, burdock root, Jerusalem artichokes, and onions, provide compounds that feed these bacteria, allowing them to flourish. In addition, whole plant foods, such as beans and whole grains, provide soluble fibers that regulate bowel function, bind to cholesterol and toxins, and slow the release of sugars into our bloodstream. As the prime spot for both the absorption of nutrients and elimination of wastes, taking care of your intestines is a key to optimal health.

2. **Decrease Cellular Damage**

Whole foods offer potent plant chemicals (phytochemicals) that decrease the negative effects free radicals have on the body. Free radicals are unstable molecules that are toxic to our cells because they attack them at the molecular level, causing destruction, mutations, and cell death. Free radical damage can contribute to cancer, heart disease, arthritis, and many other diseases. Diet is considered to be one of the most important lifestyle factors in the development of chronic disease. Phytochemicals work within the body to prevent cell mutation while keeping cells reproducing normally.

3. **Support Optimum Organ Function**

Whole foods work together to support the entire human body. Because whole foods are unprocessed, they retain all of their nutrients and fibers. Whole foods contain all of the nutrients that are needed for optimum liver function. Your liver is an important organ in detoxification. Supporting it helps to maintain a healthy weight, keeps inflammation in check, and slows down the development of many chronic diseases. Brain function also is well supported by eating whole foods. A 2006 article in neurology found that eating fresh vegetables, particularly dark, leafy greens, helps to keep the brain young, improves memory, and slows the mental decline that is sometimes associated with growing old by 40%. When it comes to cardiovascular health, a diet rich in beans, whole grains, raw nuts, and plenty of fruits and vegetables has comparable benefits to many cardiovascular medications.

4. Decrease Systemic Inflammation

A healthy body needs low amounts of inflammation. Problems arise when you take in large amounts of factory-fed animal products, refined sugar, refined vegetable oils, and refined carbohydrates. These foods have the ability to increase pain, swelling, and cellular damage. When you are in a state of chronic inflammation, it can cause chronic diseases like arthritis, heart disease, skin disorders, diabetes, obesity, high blood pressure, osteoporosis, and various cancers. When you consume an anti-inflammatory diet, or one that comes mainly from unrefined plant foods, your body produces chemicals that cause mild, rather than excessive, inflammatory reactions, which are conducive to health.

5. Assist with Hormonal Balance

To produce and metabolize hormones, our bodies need the proper ingredients. Estrogen, testosterone, and even the active form of vitamin D come from cholesterol. If our liver is functioning well, we produce all the necessary cholesterol-based hormones and still have normal cholesterol levels. Did you know that our liver also breaks down and transforms hormones when we are done with them? For example, let's look at estrogen. The liver has three choices when transforming the different forms of estrogen. It can transform estrogen into a helpful molecule, a harmful molecule, or a very harmful molecule. When we have certain foods in our diets, such as cabbage, broccoli, cauliflower, Brussels sprouts, flaxseeds, kudzu, green leafy vegetables, and beans, we transform estrogen into the beneficial form that protects our bodies. This is particularly important for women at risk of estrogen-positive cancers of the breast.

6. Regulate the Immune System

Over 50% of your immune cells are located in your intestines, with over 70% of the body's antibodies being produced there! By eating plants rich in fibers that feed beneficial bacteria, you ensure a calm environment for the first stage of your immune system. According to some researches, our intestines actually sense when certain bacteria are present. If the intestines are out of balance, chemicals are sent throughout the body, alerting other immune cells that there is a state of alarm. These alarm chemicals can increase our risk for the disease. Additionally, our immune cells need to be fed just like any other cell in the body. Many of us take vitamin C to boost our immunity and decrease the intensity and duration of a cold. Eating whole foods ensures a diet rich in vitamins A, C, and E, and the minerals zinc and selenium, which are all essential for optimum immune cell function.

7. Maintain a Healthy Weight

Food is so much more than the calories it contains. It is a complex, life-giving substance rich in nutrients and phytochemicals that acts in our bodies to change the way our genes are expressed. Quality is the most important factor in any healthy diet and weight loss plan, not quantity. By eating a whole foods diet, you ensure you are getting the highest-quality foods possible and all of the nutrients you need to maintain proper functioning of vital organs.

In addition, cutting calories too severely can send your body into a state of alarm, which increases your cortisol levels, telling your body to store fat. Instead of depriving yourself to reach an ideal weight and state of health, why not nourish yourself? Depriving yourself of nutritious food and calories activates something called neuropeptide Y in your brain, which tells you to search for food. It is highest in the morning, which makes sense after a night's fast. After a nutrient-dense meal, your stomach secretes a special chemical that shuts down appetite and stimulates the sensation of pleasure in a part of your brain. If you don't feel satisfied after a meal, then your body secretes neuropeptide Y to eat more food! Listen to your body's cues for hunger and honor them. Eating foods in their whole form helps to bring on that sense of satisfaction after a meal. It will also begin to reset your body's natural state of balance to bring on your ideal weight and optimal state of health step by step.

What are the 30 Days of Whole Food?

People eat a lot of processed foods these days. Busy people tend to eat more commercially manufactured drinks, meals, and snacks during the week. When unrestrained, these unhealthy eating habits lead to unintentional weight gain. Many chronic illnesses are influenced by an imbalanced diet and a sluggish lifestyle.

Unhealthy eating habits plus little or no exercise are major contributors to lifelong illnesses and shortened life expectancy. Luckily for you, you can reset your system by adding more whole foods to your diet and cutting your daily intake of processed food and drinks for at least 30 days.

There are a lot of diets on how to be healthy – from veganism to the ketogenic diet, to Weight Watchers, to the Atkins diet. The 30 day whole food diet is a revolutionary dietary pattern that can reset your relationship with food. The philosophy is to strictly restrict certain products without keeping track of calories and without recording the weight on the scale.

Rules for the 30 Day of Whole Food Diet:

1. **Say "yes" to real food**

Shop on the perimeter of the grocery store. Read all labels and do not buy anything with ingredients that you cannot pronounce or do not know what it actually is. Recognize every ingredient.

2. **Buy organic and grass-fed**

This isn't necessary because it is not feasible for everyone. However, if able, it helps in eliminating pesticides and GMOs from your diet.

3. **Limit processed foods**

If you absolutely have to buy something from a package, make sure you recognize every ingredient (see rule 1). To keep it simple, do not purchase anything with more than five ingredients. When purchasing processed meats, make sure that they do not have added sugar, MSG, sulfite, or carrageen.

4. **No sugar**

You will conquer your sweet tooth this month. No sugar means no sugar or sugar substitutes, maple syrup, honey, agave, nectar, coconut sugar, date syrup, stevia, Splenda, equal, NutraSweet, xylitol, etc. If you are unsure, then leave it out. If you have a sweet craving, reach for a cup of tea or fresh fruit. Even dark chocolate is out, unless you're sucking down 100% cocoa.

5. **Yes to healthy fats**

For cooking, use pastured or 100% grass-fed and organic whenever possible. Cook in animal fats, clarified butter, ghee, coconut oil, and extra-virgin olive oil. Eat avocado, cashews, coconut butter, coconut meat & flakes, canned coconut milk, hazelnuts, macadamia nuts, macadamia butter, and olives. Occasionally treat yourself to almonds, almond butter, pecans, and pistachios, but limit flax seeds, pine nuts, pumpkin seeds, sesame seeds, sunflower seeds, sunflower seed butter, and walnuts.

6. **No dairy**

Use ghee or clarified butter. Do not use regular butter as it contains milk proteins and will affect results.

7. **Yes to "pod" legumes, no to every other legume**

This means you can eat green beans, sugar snap peas, and snow peas. You cannot have beans, soy, chickpeas, peanuts, etc.

8. **No alcohol or tobacco products**
9. **A "Yes, I can" attitude. Believe in your success from day one!**

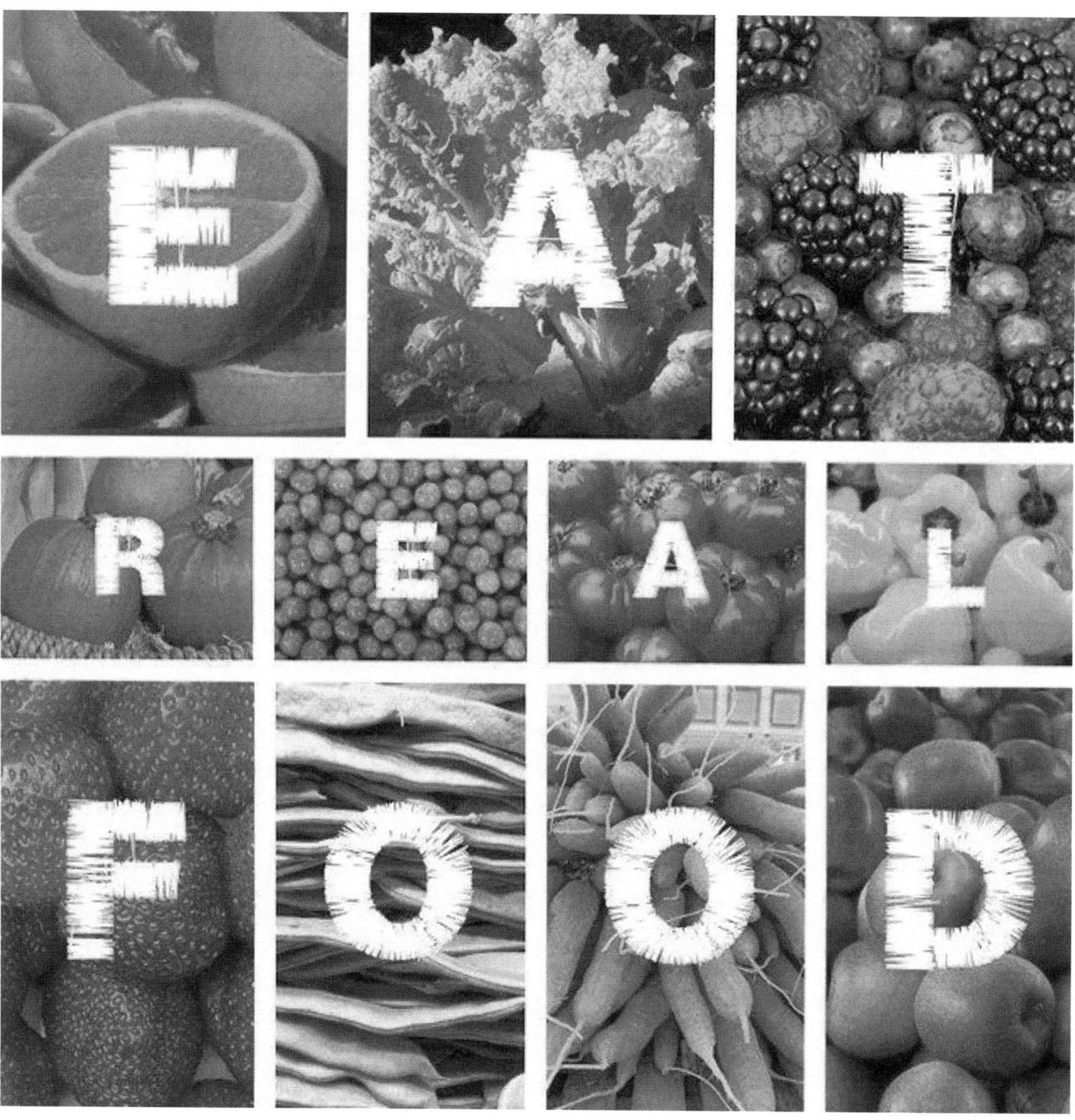

Foods to Eat

Below you can find a list of delicious whole foods that are unprocessed or minimally processed that you can enjoy without guilt during the month-long challenge.

Stock your refrigerator and pantry by grocery shopping with the full shopping list below:

Vegetables: All vegetables are allowed – including potatoes! Here's a full list of all the encouraged vegetables:

- Potatoes
- Asparagus
- Green beans
- Romaine lettuce
- Broccoli
- Bell pepper
- Carrot
- Red bell pepper
- Tomatoes
- Olives
- Avocado
- Garlic
- Cabbage
- Cucumber
- Brussels sprout
- Iceberg lettuce
- Celery
- Spinach
- Onion
- Zucchini
- Jalapeno peppers
- Pumpkin
- Sweet potatoes
- Peas
- Artichoke
- Mushrooms
- Kale
- Spinach
- Ginger
- Beets
- Eggplants
- Collard greens
- Chives
- Fennel
- Okra
- Leeks
- Radishes

Meat and Poultry: Unprocessed meat and poultry are allowed during 30 days of whole food, but be attentive to added sugars and processed meats. Go shopping for these kinds of meat and poultry:

- Beef
- Ground beef
- Beef heart
- Beef Liver
- Beef tongue
- Buffalo, bison
- Goat
- Rabbit
- Mutton
- Chicken
- Lamb
- Pork
- Ham
- Ribs
- Pork shoulder
- Veal
- Bacon
- Burger
- Duck
- Duck Liver
- Chicken liver
- Turkey
- Quail
- Pheasant

Fruits: Both fresh and dried fruits are allowed during the 30 days of whole food, this includes:

- Bananas
- Apples

- Oranges
- Mangos
- Watermelon
- Pineapples
- Papaya
- Grapefruit
- Pomegranate
- Pear
- Peach
- Plum
- Grapes
- Kiwi
- Strawberries
- Blueberries
- Lemons
- Limes

Fish and Seafood: Fish and shellfish are encouraged, including:

- Tilapia
- Salmon
- Tuna
- Trout
- Black Cod
- Halibut
- Cod
- Catfish
- Barramundi
- Arctic char
- Crab
- Lobster
- Shrimp
- Clams
- Mussels
- Oysters
- Scallops

Fats:

- Coconut oil
- Avocado oil
- Sesame oil
- Sunflower oil
- Canola oil
- Olive oil
- Ghee (clarified butter)
- Lard
- Duck fat
- Almond butter

Nuts and seeds: All nuts and seeds are encouraged during the 30 days of whole food with the exception of peanuts, this includes:

- Nut milk (almond milk, cashew milk, flax milk, hazelnut milk, etc.)
- Nut flours (almond flour, coconut flour, flaxseed meal, macadamia nut
- flour, pistachio flour, cashew nut flour, etc.)
- Almonds
- Cashews
- Chestnuts
- Pecans
- Walnuts
- Pine nuts
- Macadamia nuts
- Flaxseeds
- Sesame seeds
- Chia seeds
- Sunflower seeds
- Pumpkin seeds

Vinegar:

- White vinegar
- Red wine vinegar
- Balsamic vinegar
- Apple cider vinegar

Herbs and seasonings: To enhance the flavors of your meal, there are no restrictions on seasonings, spices, and herbs.

Foods to Avoid

During your 30 days of whole food, there is some food that is restricted. It's extremely important you don't have any cheat days or sneak in any of these foods in your meals for your success.

Dairy: Dairy is not recommended during the 30 days whole food, whether its full-fat or low-fat. The only exception of dairy allowed is ghee. Items to avoid include:

- Butter
- Milk
- Whey, milk powder
- Ice cream
- Frozen desserts
- Yogurt
- Soy and soy products

- Cottage cheese
- Sour cream
- Dips
- Natural and processed cheese
- Butter
- Non-dairy coffee creamer

Alcohol: No alcohol in any form is allowed, whether it's for cooking or drinking. This includes:

- Beer
- Tequila
- Vodka

- Gin
- Rum
- Vanilla extract

Note: The closest thing to alcohol is cooking vinegar, such as red wine vinegar, white vinegar, apple cider vinegar, etc.

Grains: All grains must be avoided, including:

- Rice
- Quinoa
- Oats
- Barley
- Maze
- Wheat

- Millet
- Farro
- Rye
- Buckwheat
- Spelt

Legumes: Legumes must be avoided, the only exceptions are peas and green beans. Avoid the following:

- Tofu
- Soy sauce
- Miso
- Edamame

- Chickpeas
- Lentils
- Peanuts

Sugar and sweeteners: Sugar of any form is absolutely restricted. This includes sweeteners such as Swerve, Splenda, etc.

Processed additives: Any foods that contain MSG, carrageenan, or sulfites must be avoided.

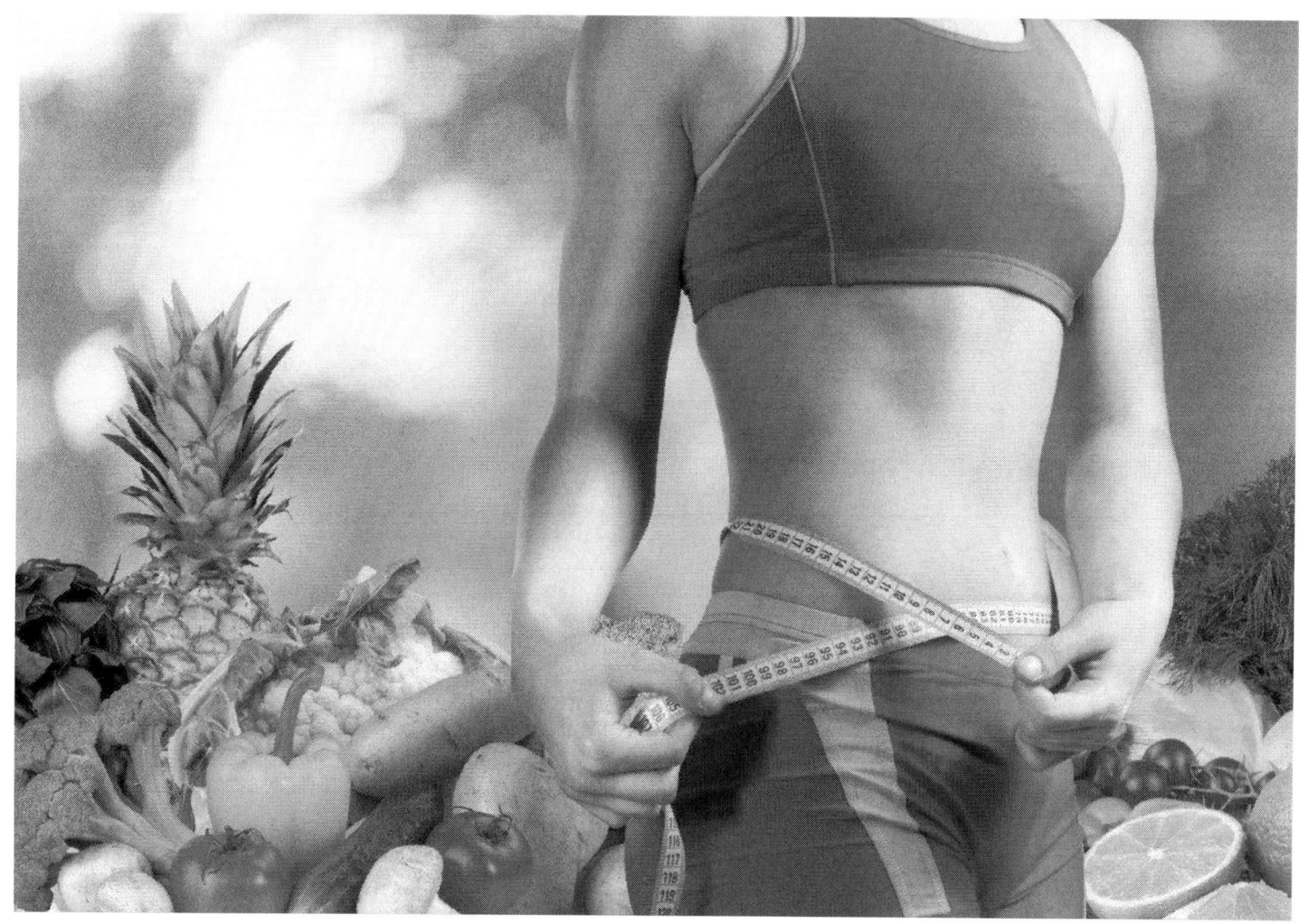

Tips for the Whole Food Diet

Adopting a new diet can be sometimes difficult. However, with these tips, you can certainly survive the 30 days whole food diet.

- ✓ **Get enough sleep**

Sleep is often an underestimated aspect of a diet. However, sleep is crucial as it allows your body to heal. Your metabolism and sleep are controlled by the same centers of your brain. Sleep deprivation can lead to weight gain. Do your best to improve your quality of sleep, and you will certainly feel better and motivated.

- ✓ **Drink enough water**

Water is the essential substance in your body so you must remain hydrated. You should drink approximately 10 glasses of water daily and remain well hydrated during the 30 days. Drinking enough water allows your liver to break down fats more effectively. You most likely will need additional water to make up for caffeinated beverages you eliminated from your diet.

- ✓ **Exercise**

To meet your goals, exercising is important. Exercising helps increases muscle function and reduces the fat content in your body. You can choose between cardio, strength, or flexibility exercises, which can give you enough physical activity daily to improve and maintain a healthy body.

✓ **Eat more vegetables**

Adding vegetables to your meals increases the nutritious value. For instance, eat vegetables as sides or as part of the main entrée. Examples include:

- Add spinach, onions, and herbs to egg omelets
- Puree carrots or other vegetables in smoothies
- Mix cauliflower or broccoli into scrambled eggs
- Try butternut squash pancakes than regular flour pancakes.
- Add zucchini or spinach to homemade brownies
- Add extra vegetables to soups and stews
- Serve your favorite vegetables along with chicken, beef, pork, and fish recipes.

✓ **Substitute foods**

You can replace processed foods with some whole foods. Such examples include:

- Coconut aminos instead of tamari and soy sauce
- Coconut flour instead of all-purpose flour
- Flax meal instead of breadcrumbs
- Unsweetened coconut or almont milk instead of cow's milk
- Lettuc instead of using bread
- Cauliflower rice instead of rice
- Fresh vegetables instead of canned vegetables
- Spiralized squash or zucchini instead of pasta noodles
- Unsweetened plain Greek yogurt with fruit instead of branded yogurt
- Frozen unsweetened smoothies instead of ice cream

✓ **Plan your meals ahead**

You might become tired and don't feel like cooking anything, especially since whole foods are more time consuming than processed and packaged dishes. The answer is to plan your meals. This can mean doing all the food preparation for the recipe before dinnertime or have a simple lettuce salad stored in your refrigerator.

✓ **Do not be afraid of mistakes**

You aren't a robot who can just be reprogrammed to eat only whole foods, so don't expect a success without making some mistakes. You may accidentally eat or drink something you shouldn't have, and you must be prepared to forgive yourself. Being prepared for mistakes will make you feel less guilty when you drink a can of Coca-Cola or eat that chocolate chip cookie.

✓ **Find an accountability partner**

Some people cannot motivate themselves during the 30 days. The support and validation from other people are encouraged, whether it's from friends or family. It can be reassuring to know that you can talk to someone when you're having a tough day and someone who understands the challenges you are facing.

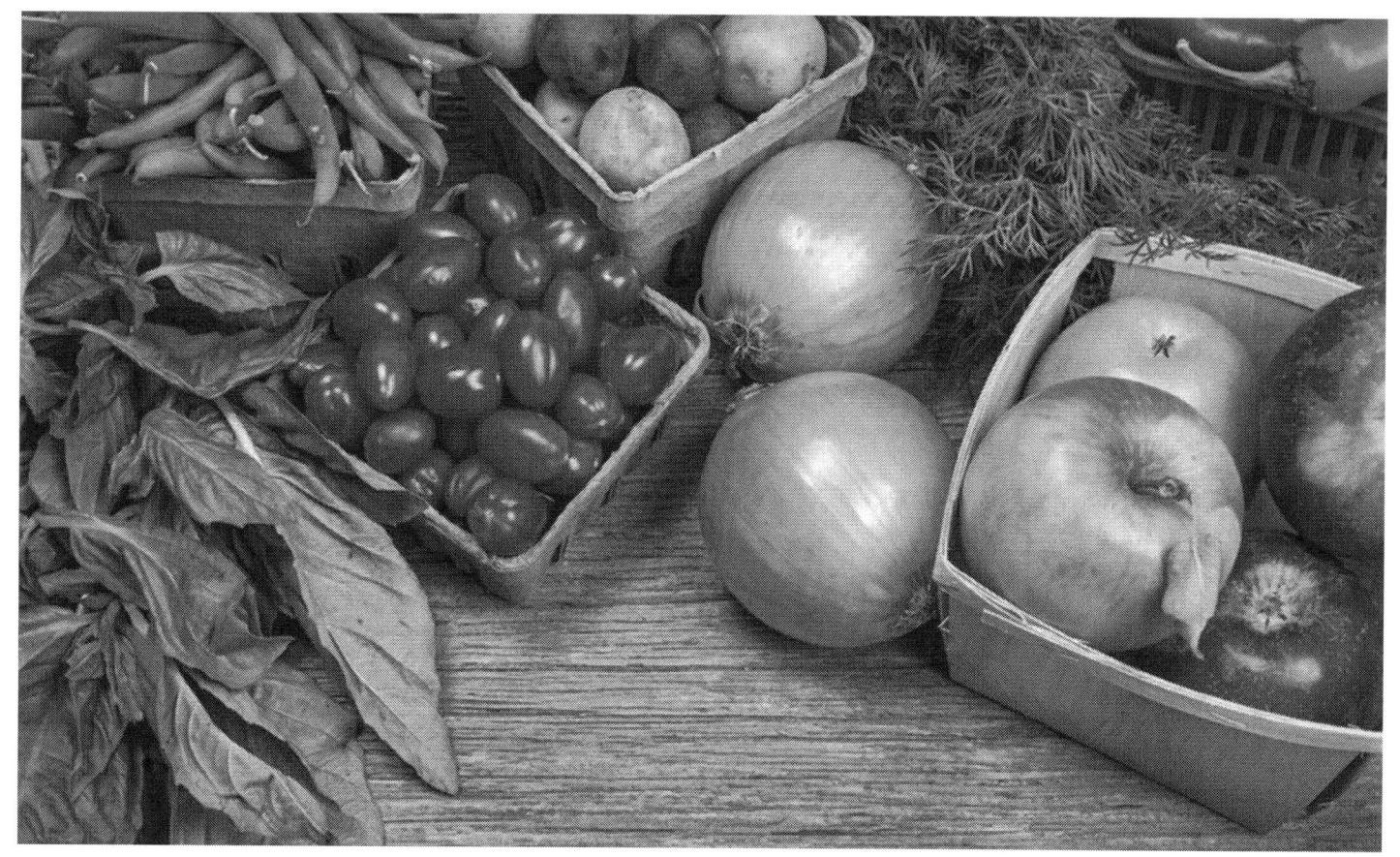

The Essential Five

1. Berries

Berries are nature's sweetest and most delicious offerings—and they're exceptionally good for you as well. The term berry is used in it's colloquial rather than its scientific form, including cherries, grapes, cranberries, currants, and so on. It is recommended that you eat berries regularly— perhaps every day if you enjoy them. If you have a sweet tooth, they can be a replacement for processed, sugary sweets.

Scientific evidences support the health benefits of berries. Berries have been shown to potentially protect against cancer. They also appear to protect against cognitive decline. Studies have found that consuming berries daily lowers blood pressure, a factor associated with a lower risk of cardiovascular disease. These benefits may be due to the high antioxidant content of these small but powerful fruits, as berries contain more antioxidants per serving than any other food except spices.

Some people worry that berries (and fruits in general) are a sugary food that should be avoided, causing diabetes and weight gain. But these fears are misguided. Yes, berries and other fruits contain high levels of fructose, but when it comes in the form of whole fruit, with plentiful fiber and water, fructose has a different effect on the body than it does in its isolated, highly processed forms.

So go ahead and add some fresh berries to your breakfast bowl, together with cereal like oatmeal. If you drink smoothies, a small handful of berries adds a boost of sweetness, a good companion for lots of greens. Berries also make a wonderful enhancement to a salad. Throw them in whole or blend a handful of raspberries with some white balsamic vinegar for a delicious, oil-free raspberry vinaigrette.

Choose organic berries when possible because conventional varieties often contain an unhealthy dose of pesticides. Frozen berries are a good choice, retaining all the health benefits of the fresh fruit. Be careful with dried berries, such as raisins, dried currants, goji berries, or dried cranberries—although still a healthy choice, the loss of water concentrates them, making them more calorie-dense. Eat them in limited quantities, especially if weight loss is a goal.

2. Beans and Other Legumes

As you shift to a whole foods, you are likely to eat many more of these nourishing foods and enjoy the many benefits, hopefully daily. If you're concerned that it might get monotonous, don't be—this group of foods comprises more than thirteen hundred varieties of beans, peas, and lentils.

The legume family includes all the varieties of dried or cooked beans you can find at grocery stores: black, pinto, navy, cannellini, kidney, garbanzo (also known as chickpeas), black-eyed peas, and so on. Legumes are generally low-fat, high-protein, starchy foods packed with vitamins, minerals, antioxidant compounds, and dietary fiber. As you shift to a 90% and higher plant-based diet, you will find that these highly satiating foods are a great replacement for some of the meat you are accustomed to eating, offering many of the same beneficial nutrients without the cholesterol and saturated fat, and with the added fiber and other micronutrients found only in plant foods. Almost all varieties of legumes provide iron, zinc, B vitamins, magnesium, and potassium, among many other nutrients.

3. Leafy Greens

Researchers at Harvard University found greens to be the food most highly associated with protection from major chronic disease and cardiovascular disease. They also reduce the risk of diabetes. Greens are packed with fiber, protein, and antioxidants, as well as a long list of vitamins, minerals, and disease-fighting phytochemicals.

You can eat greens raw, toss them into soup or stew, blend them into flavorful pesto-style sauces, add steamed greens to mashed potatoes, or water-sauté them with garlic. Spinach is a nutrient-rich addition to homemade hummus or other bean spreads. Try to eat greens every day.

4. Nonstarchy Vegetables

Only one in ten Americans eats enough fruits and vegetables. If Americans ate just one more serving of fruits and vegetables daily, it would save more than thirty thousand lives annually, and billions of dollars in medical costs. No matter how many points nutritionists and dietary experts seem to argue about, this is the one that they universally agree upon: eat more vegetables! Eat the rainbow. Colorful vegetables tend to contain the most antioxidants, and where antioxidants go, health tends to follow. Brighten your plate and eat as many different color as possible.

5. Nuts and Seeds

Nuts and seeds round out our list of essential whole foods to enjoy daily. We feel these are an important category of foods for many reasons. The simplest, of course, is that nuts and seeds are packed with health-promoting nutrients and are consistently associated with good health outcomes. Nuts and seeds are considered to reduce the risk of heart disease and diabetes, as well as increase life span.

This category of food also contains some of the most concentrated plant sources of essential omega-3 fatty acids. The body cannot make these important nutrients, so we have to get them from food or supplements. Although many whole plant foods contain small amounts of omega-3 fatty acids, some nuts and seeds, such as flaxseeds, chia seeds, hemp seeds, and walnuts, contain particularly high amounts.

Nuts and seeds can easily be mixed into your favorite foods. Sprinkle a few chopped almonds on morning oatmeal or add them to salads. Nuts can be blended with fresh herbs to make a salad dressing or creamy pesto. Ground flaxseeds or hemp seed are easily added to smoothies, sprinkled over breakfast cereal or oatmeal, or baked in muffins. Flaxseeds and chia seeds have a "binding" quality, and are ideal for thickening sauces or replacing eggs in baking.

Setting Up a Whole Food Kitchen and Pantry

Imagine starting the 30 day whole food diet and then coming home to a kitchen full of unhealthy processed food such as pancake and chocolate brownie mixes, potato chips, and ice cream. Naturally, every single day would be a struggle. But when you have a kitchen and pantry that promote the whole food diet, your life will be so much easier. You do not have to spend a lot of money to convert your kitchen into a healthy one.

Check your fridge and pantry

What have you got inside your refrigerator? With a box at your side, open up its doors and start purging all processed, unhealthy foods. Do the exact same thing to your pantry.

After this, make a list of all the substitutes you will need for the food items that you got rid of. For instance, if you had to give up your diet cola, then substitute it with green tea or lemon water. That means you need to buy a lemon and then constantly fill up a glass pitcher with water to put lemon slices in it. Store it in the fridge and reach for it each time you have the urge for a soda.

Stock up on whole food staples

Giving up certain common food does not mean you have to suffer through tasteless meals. In fact, doing this will buy you a one-way ticket back to your former diet. Invest in quality sea salt, black pepper, olive oil, coconut oil, herbs and spices, nuts and seeds, coconut milk, organic eggs, fresh greens, meats, seafood, fruit, and other staples that you need.

This will be easier if you make it a habit to plan your meals ahead and make a grocery list that will guide you at the store. You can use the recipes in the succeeding chapters to prepare your meal plans.

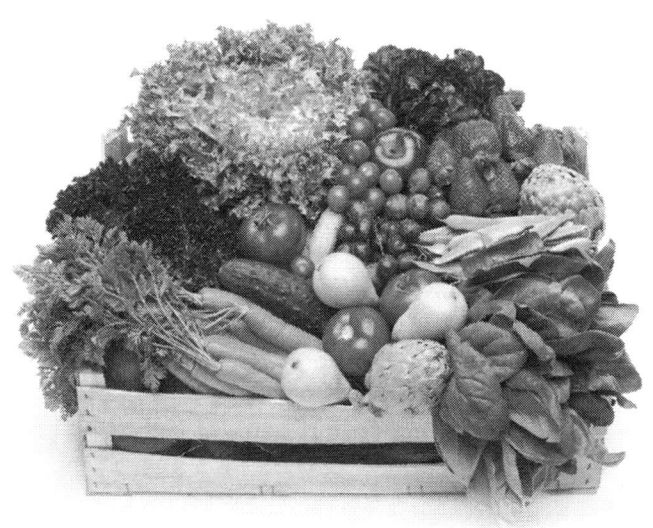

Chapter 2. Recipes

BREAKFAST

Oatmeal Fruit Shake

Prep time: 10 minutes

Cooking time: none

Servings: 2

Nutrients per serving:

Carbohydrates – 58 g

Fat – 1.5 g

Protein – 5 g

Calories – 270

Ingredients:

- 1 cup oatmeal, already prepared and cooled
- 1 apple, cored and roughly chopped
- 1 banana, halved
- 1 cup baby spinach
- 2 cups coconut water
- 2 cups ice, cubed
- ½ tsp ground cinnamon
- 1 tsp pure vanilla extract

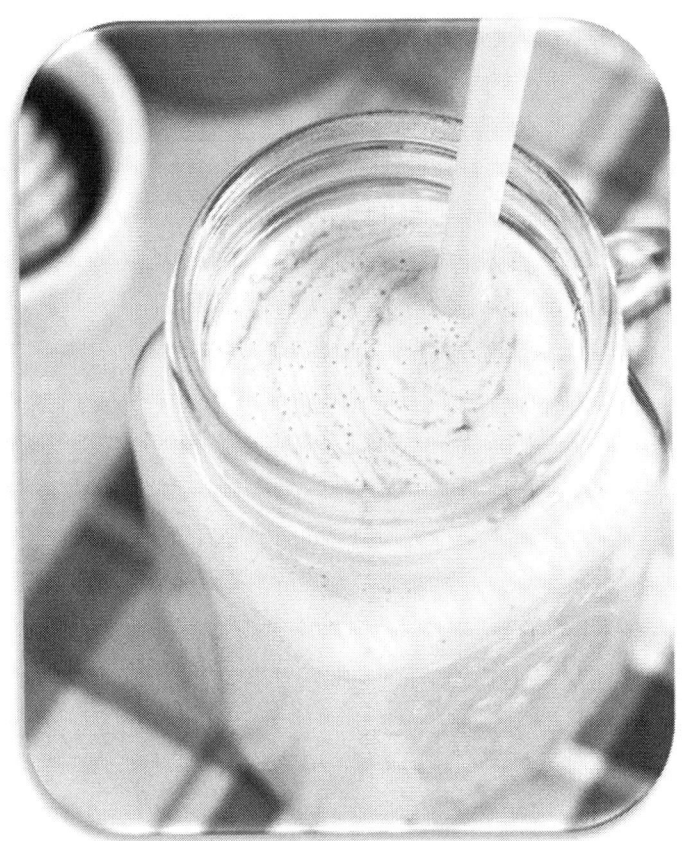

Instructions:

1. Add all ingredients to blender.
2. Blend from low to high for several minutes until smooth.

Pumpkin Pie Smoothie

Prep time: 5 minutes

Cooking time: none

Servings: 2

Nutrients per serving:

Carbohydrates – 30 g

Fat – 2.5 g

Protein – 5 g

Calories – 150

Ingredients:

- 1 cup pumpkin puree
- 1 large ripe banana
- 1 cup unsweetened soy milk
- 2 pitted dates
- ½ tsp pure vanilla extract
- 1¼ tsp pumpkin pie spice
- 5 ice cubes
- ½ tsp ground flaxseeds
- Pinch of nutmeg

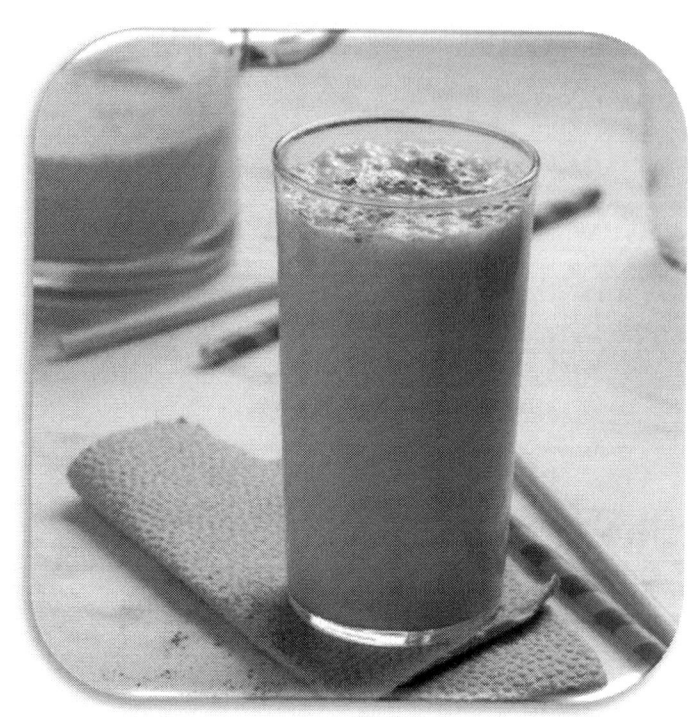

Instructions:

1. Mix all ingredients in a blender and blend until smooth.

Breakfast Green Machine Smoothie

Prep time: 5 minutes

Cooking time: none

Servings: 2

Nutrients per serving:

Carbohydrates – 29 g

Fat – 8 g

Protein – 8 g

Calories – 210

Ingredients:

- 1 medium cucumber, peeled and chopped
- 2-3 leaves green kale
- ½ cup baby spinach
- 1 banana
- ½ cup frozen mango
- 3 Tbsp hemp hearts
- 1 tsp matcha
- 1 cup unsweetened nondairy milk of your choice

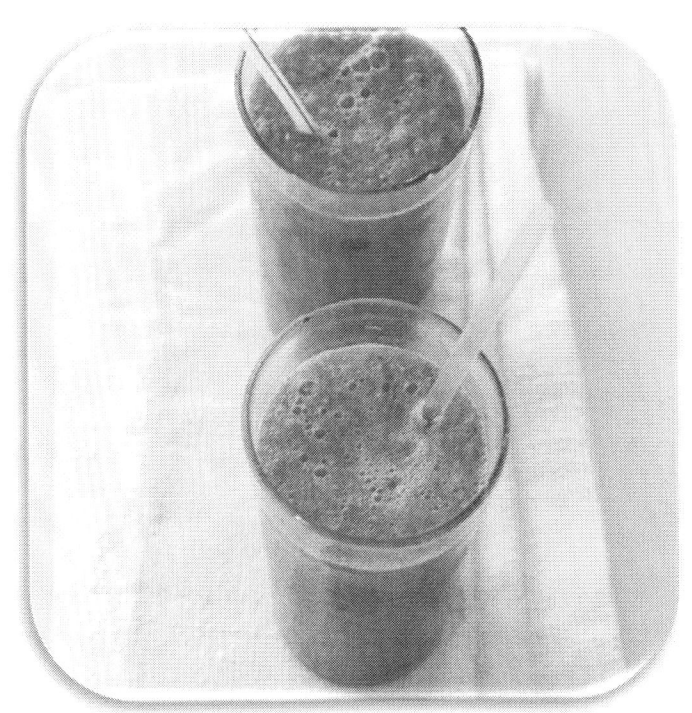

Instruction:

1. Mix all ingredients in a blender until smooth.

Breakfast Sandwich

Prep time: 15 minutes

Cooking time: 20 minutes

Servings: 4

Nutrients per serving:

Carbohydrates – 21 g

Fat – 21 g

Protein – 18 g

Calories – 340

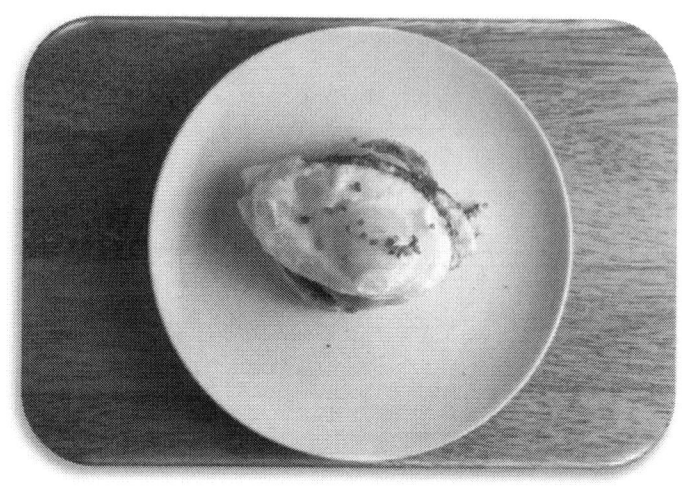

Ingredients:

- 2 Tbsp extra-virgin olive oil, divided
- ¾ cup yellow onion, chopped
- 2 garlic cloves, chopped
- ¾ Tsp sea salt, divided
- 1 ¾ cup mashed potatoes
- ¼ tsp black pepper
- 4 patties breakfast sausage, prepared
- 4 eggs, poached

Instruction:

1. Heat half of the oil in a skillet. Sauté the onion, garlic, and a quarter teaspoon of salt until the onion is golden brown, around six to eight minutes. Combine this mix with the potatoes, pepper, and the rest of the salt. Shape into four 4-inch patties.
2. Heat the remaining oil in the skillet and cook the patties, carefully flipping them so they're golden on both sides. This should take about ten minutes. Put them onto plates, top with the sausage, an egg, and serve.

Veggie and Tofu Scramble

Prep time: 15 minutes

Cooking time: 8 minutes

Servings: 4

Nutrients per serving:

Carbohydrates – 7 g

Fat – 7 g

Protein – 12 g

Calories – 120

Ingredients:

- 2 cups lightly packed spinach leaves
- 1 large tomato, quartered
- ½ red or yellow bell pepper, quartered
- ½ red onion, quartered
- 3 cloves garlic
- 1 (14-ounce) package firm tofu, well drained
- ⅛ tsp fine sea salt

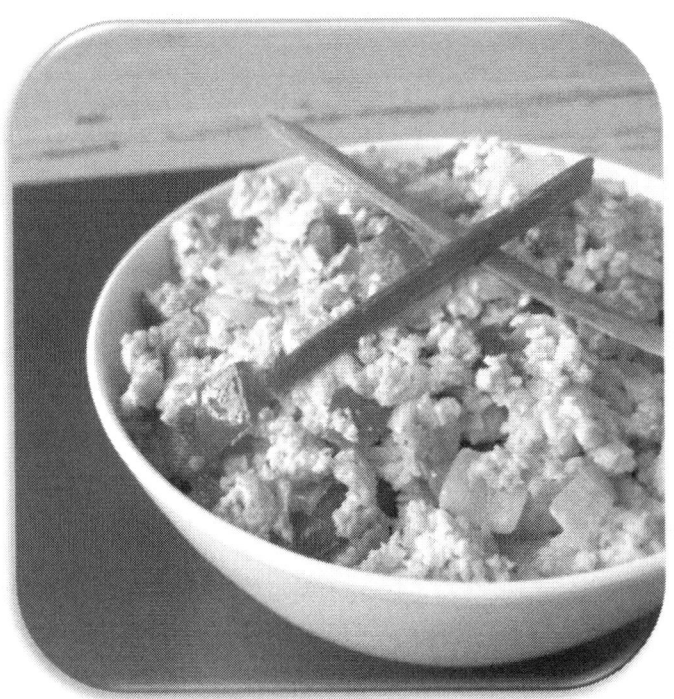

Instruction:

1. In a food processor, combine first five ingredients and pulse until finely chopped.
2. Put vegetable mixture in a skillet over medium-high heat and bring to a simmer. Crumble in tofu and sprinkle with salt. Cook, until most of the liquid has evaporated, about 8 minutes. Serve warm.

Breakfast Banana Splits

Prep time: 15 minutes

Cooking time: none

Servings: 8

Nutrients per serving:

Carbohydrates – 49 g

Fat – 3 g

Protein – 6 g

Calories – 250

Ingredients:

- 1 banana, halved lengthwise
- 1 blueberry & pomegranate Greek yogurt
- ½ cup breakfast cereal
- ¼ cup trail mix

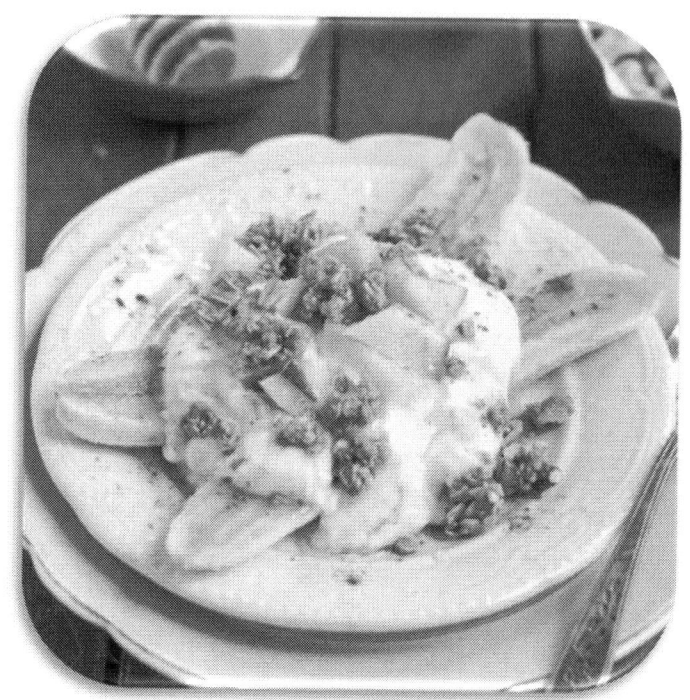

Instruction:

1. Arrange banana halves in a bowl. Top with the yogurt, drizzle of fruit sauce, trail mix, and cereal to serve.

Whole Wheat Blueberry Pancakes

Prep time: 20 minutes

Cooking time: 5 minutes

Servings: 4

Nutrients per serving:

Carbohydrates – 52 g

Fat – 2 g

Protein – 4 g

Calories – 260

Ingredients:

- 2 cups whole wheat pastry flour
- 2 tsp baking powder
- 1 tsp ground cinnamon
- ¼ tsp fine sea salt
- 1 cup soy mill
- ¼ cup unsweetened applesauce
- 1 tsp pure vanilla extract
- 1¼ cups fresh or frozen blueberries

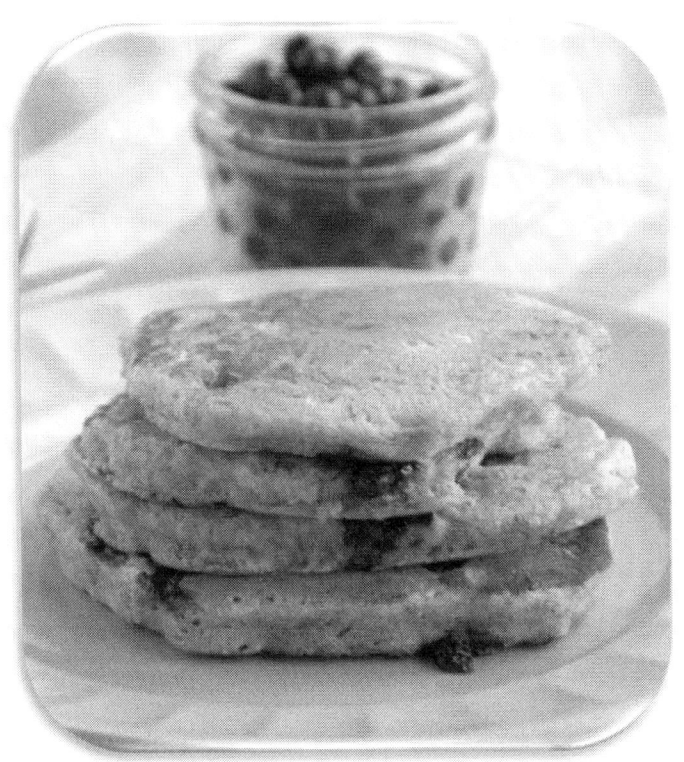

Instruction:

1. In a large bowl, whisk together first four ingredients. In a separate medium bowl, whisk together almond milk, ¼ to ½ cup water (or additional almond milk), applesauce, and vanilla until blended. Pour milk mixture into flour mixture and stir until well. Set batter aside to rest 10 minutes.
2. Heat a cast-iron griddle or nonstick skillet over medium heat until hot. Stir blueberries into batter. Ladle about ¼ cup batter onto the griddle and cook about 2 minutes. Flip and cook 1 to 2 minutes longer.

Kasha Breakfast Porridge

Prep time: 10 minutes

Cooking time: 20 minutes

Servings: 3-4

Nutrients per serving:

Carbohydrates – 39 g

Fat – 1.5 g

Protein – 5 g

Calories – 180

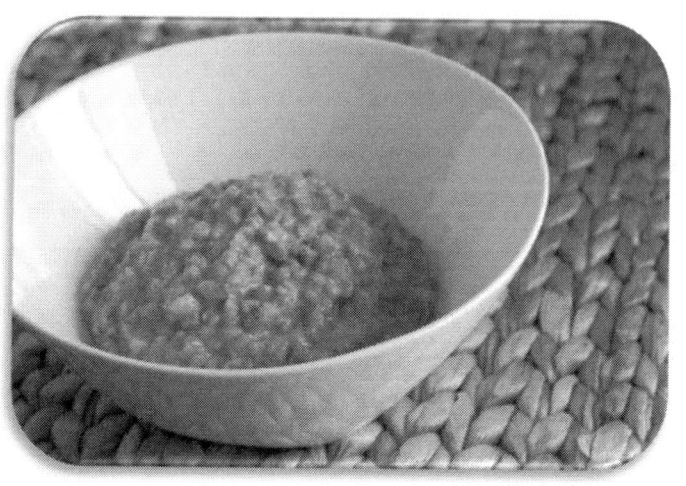

Ingredients:

- 2 cup water
- 1 stick cinnamon
- 1 cup kasha
- 1 pinch salt

Instruction:

1. In a saucepan, mix together the water and cinnamon stick and bring this to a boil.
2. Add the kasha and salt. Reduce the heat to low and cook for fifteen minutes. Serve.

Breakfast Turkey Sausage

Prep time: 10 minutes

Cooking time: 15 minutes

Servings: 8

Nutrients per serving:

Carbohydrates – 4 g

Fat – 9 g

Protein – 17 g

Calories – 170

Ingredients:

- 1 ½ lb ground turkey
- 2 apples, grated
- ½ cup flat-leaf parsley, chopped
- 3 Tbsp fresh sage, minced
- 1 ½ tsp sea salt
- ½ tsp pepper
- ½ tsp ground nutmeg
- 2 eggs, beaten
- Vegetable oil

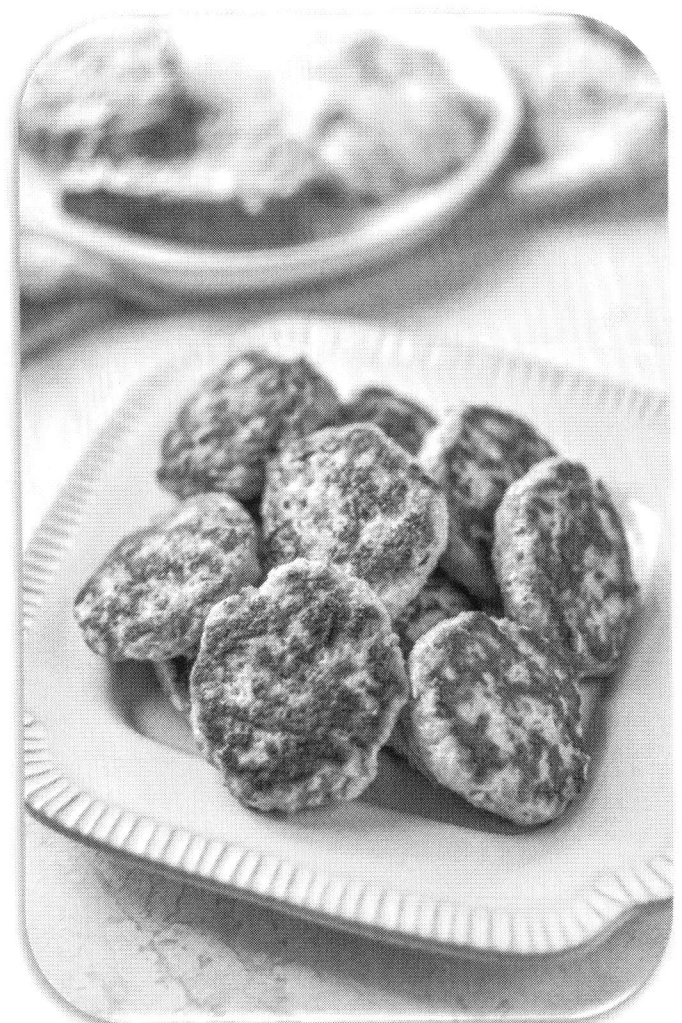

Instruction:

1. Preheat oven to 350° F.
2. Combine the turkey and eggs in a bowl. Add the rest of the ingredients. Mix well.
3. Grease a nonstick skillet with the oil.
4. Shape the sausage mix into eight patties, about a third of a cup each.
5. Brown the sausage patties for three minutes on either side. Transfer to a baking sheet and bake until the turkey has cooked, about ten minutes.

Mini Sausage Breakfast Sandwiches

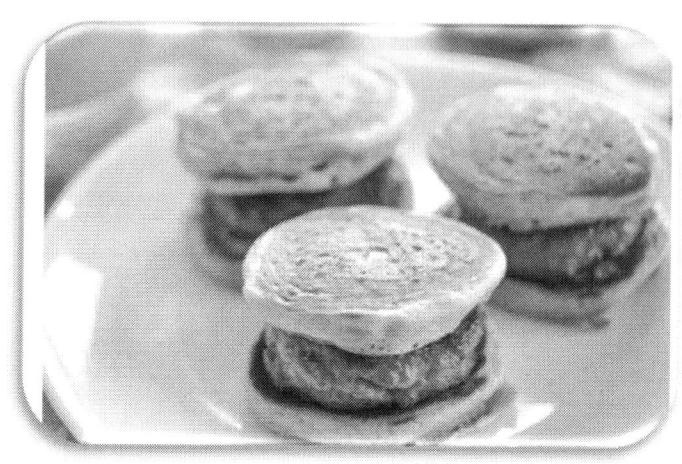

Prep time: 10 minutes

Cooking time: 4 minutes

Servings: 4

Nutrients per serving:

Carbohydrates – 40 g

Fat – 8 g

Protein – 8 g

Calories – 270

Ingredients:

- Olive oil spray
- 2 apple chicken sausages, sliced
- 32 whole wheat mini pancakes, prepared
- 3 Tbsp apple butter

Instruction:

1. Spray a skillet with oil. Cook the sausage and stir until cooked, around 3-4 minutes.
2. Put a slice of sausage on a pancake and top with the apple butter and a pancake. Serve.

Amaranth Banana Breakfast Porridge

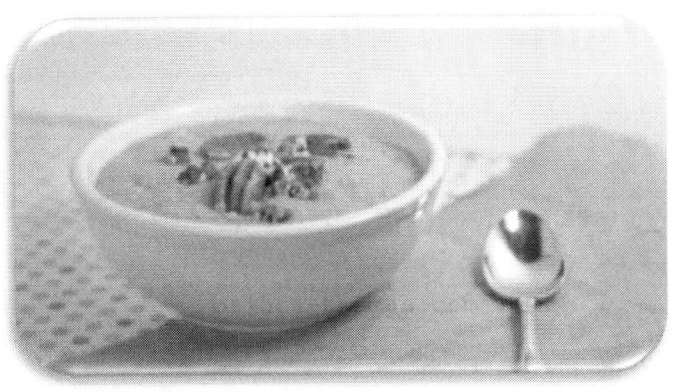

Prep time: 10 minutes

Cooking time: 25 minutes

Servings: 6-8

Nutrients per serving:

Carbohydrates – 62 g

Fat – 6 g

Protein – 10 g

Calories – 330

Ingredients:

- 2 cup amaranth
- 2 cinnamon sticks
- 4 bananas, diced
- 2 Tbsp chopped pecans
- 4 cups water

Instruction:

1. Combine the amaranth, water, and cinnamon sticks, and banana in a pot. Cover and let simmer around 25 minutes.
2. Remove from heat and discard the cinnamon. Places into bowls, and top with pecans.

Orangeade

Prep time: 15 minutes

Cooking time: 0 minutes

Servings: 4

Nutrients per serving:

Carbohydrates – 24 g

Fat – 0 g

Protein – 0.6 g

Calories – 94

Ingredients:

- 1½ cups freshly squeezed orange juice
- 3 Tbsp agave nectar
- 4 cups water

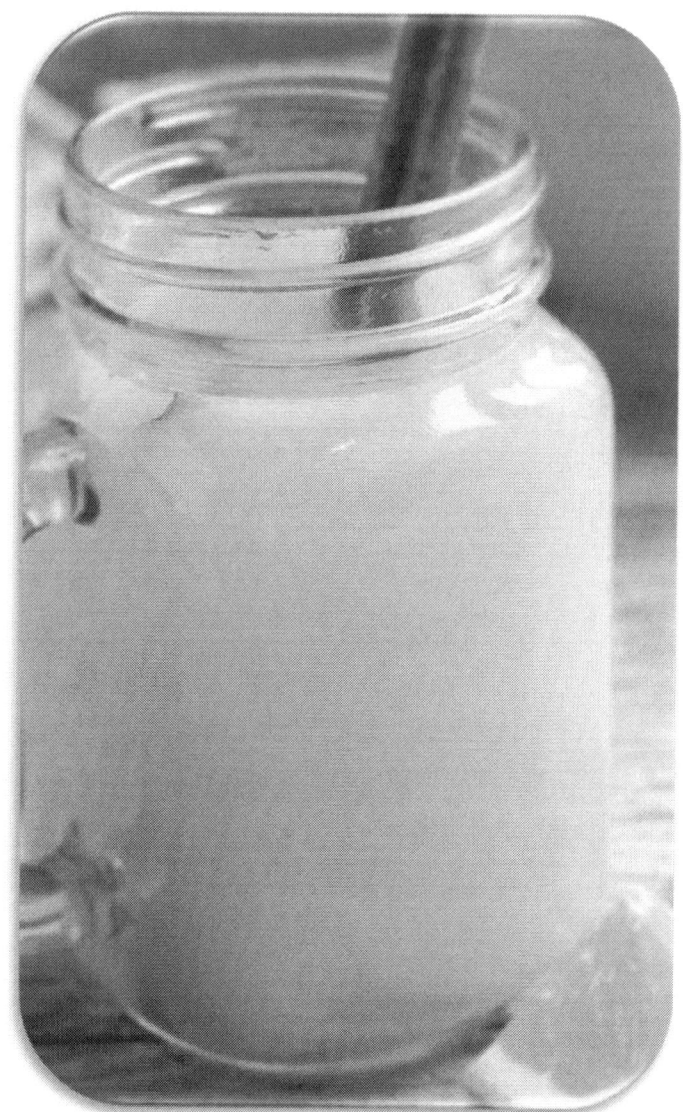

Instruction:

1. Pour all ingredients into a large pitcher. Stir until the agave nectar dissolves.

LUNCH

Deviled Ham Tea Sandwiches

Prep time: 15 minutes (+2 hours)

Cooking time: none

Servings: 6

Nutrients per serving:

Carbohydrates – 29 g

Fat – 10 g

Protein – 12 g

Calories – 250

Ingredients:

- 2 cup ham, minced
- 2 Tbsp flat-leaf parsley, minced
- 2 Tbsp green onions, minced
- 1 Tbsp Worcestershire sauce
- ¼ Ttsp chipotle sauce
- 12 sandwich bread slices

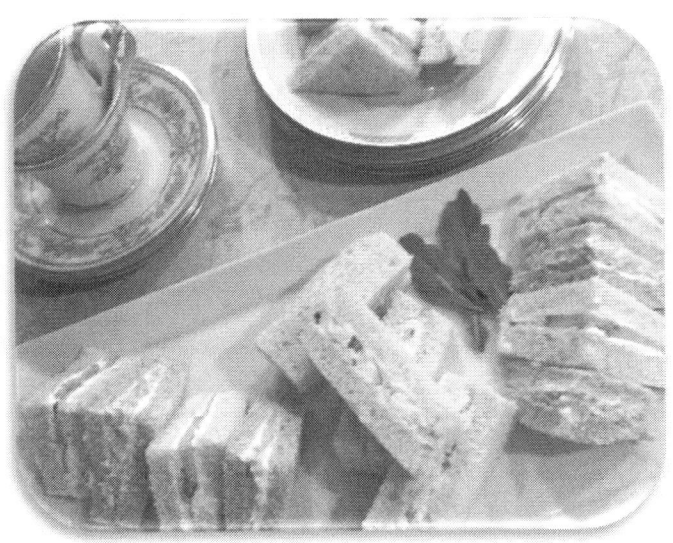

Instruction:

1. Put the ham through the sauce into a bowl and mix to cCombine all ingredients except bread. Cover and chill for 2 hours.
2. Divide the ham between the 6 slices of bread and spread out with a knife. Top with the rest of the bread and press down lightly.

Oil-Free Herb Pesto

Prep time: 25 minutes

Cooking time: none

Servings: 2

Nutrients per serving:

Carbohydrates – 3 g

Fat – 4.5 g

Protein – 2 g

Calories –60

Ingredients:

- 2 cups lightly packed basil leaves, chopped
- ¼ cup parsley, chopped
- ¼ cup leeks, chopped
- 2 cloves garlic
- ½ cup lightly dry-toasted pine nuts
- 2 Tbsp nutritional yeast
- ½ avocado, pit, skin removed
- ½ tsp coarse sea salt
- Water, as needed

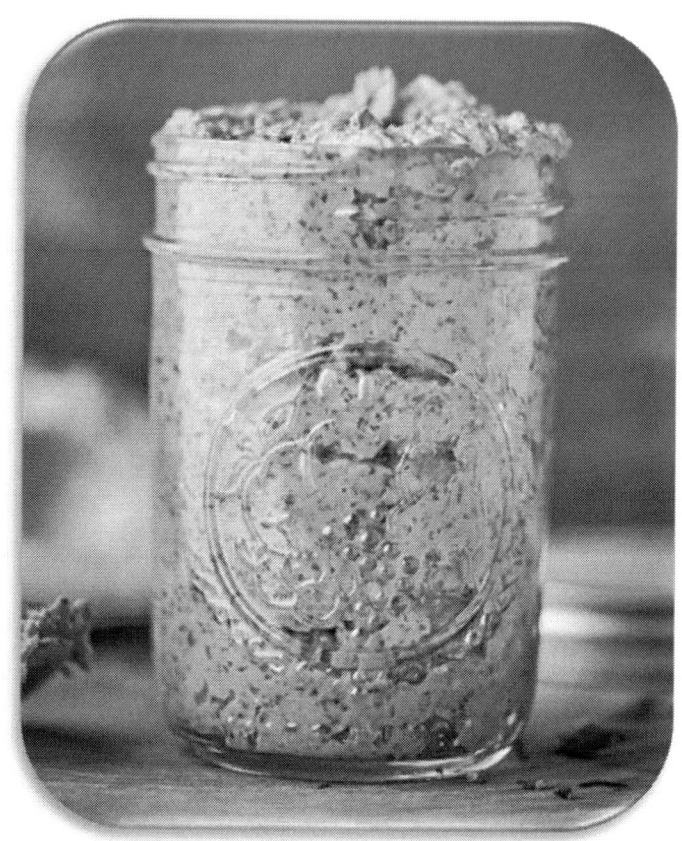

Instruction:

1. In a food processor, add all ingredients. Blend to finely minced, taking off the lid and scraping sides as needed.
2. Once the mix is finely minced, add a small amount of water and blend a bit more, leaving some texture to the mixture so it is not fully smooth.

Refried Bean and Avocado Soft Tacos

Prep time: 20 minutes

Cooking time: 20 minutes

Servings: 4

Nutrients per serving:

Carbohydrates – 64 g

Fat – 13 g

Protein – 14 g

Calories –420

Ingredients:

- 1 white onion, finely chopped
- 2 cloves garlic, minced
- 1½ cups low-sodium vegetable broth
- 2 15-oz cans no-salt-added pinto beans, drained and rinsed
- 1½ tsp cumin
- ½ tsp fine sea salt
- ¼ tsp ground black pepper
- 8 corn tortillas
- 2 cups romaine lettuce, shredded
- 3 Roma tomatoes, diced
- 1½ avocados, thinly sliced

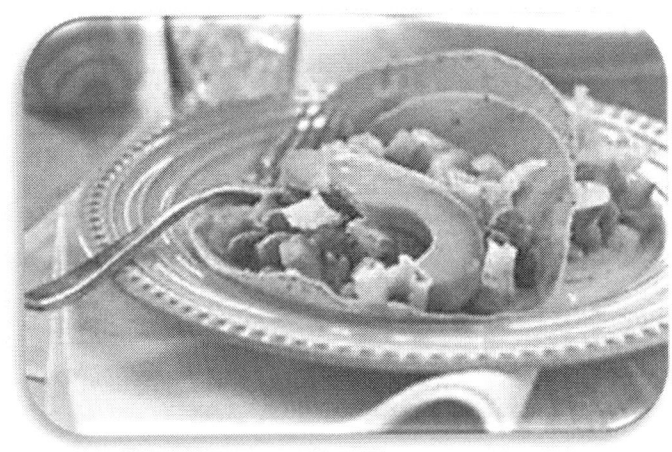

Instruction:

1. Heat a skillet over medium heat. Add onion and garlic and cook 3-4 minutes, or until they begin to stick to the skillet.
2. Stir in ½ cup broth and cook 6-8 minutes, or until onion is translucent and very tender. Reduce heat to medium-low, add beans, and cook 2-3 minutes to soften, stirring frequently.
3. Mash beans with a potato masher. Stir in remaining broth, cumin, salt, and pepper.
4. Cook 5 minutes longer, stirring occasionally and adding water or more broth as needed for desired consistency.
5. In a dry skillet over medium heat, warm each tortilla to soften. Top with a generous scoop of bean mixture. Add lettuce, tomatoes, and avocados. Fold in half and serve.

Fresh Salsa

Prep time: 10 minutes

Cooking time: none

Servings: 2

Nutrients per serving:

Carbohydrates – 6 g

Fat – 0 g

Protein – 1 g

Calories –25

Ingredients:

- 2 cups chopped tomatoes
- ⅓ cup chopped yellow or white onion
- 2 Tbsp chopped fresh cilantro
- 2 Tbsp lime juice
- 1 to 2 jalapeño or serrano peppers, stemmed, seeded, and finely chopped
- ¼ tsp fine sea salt (optional)

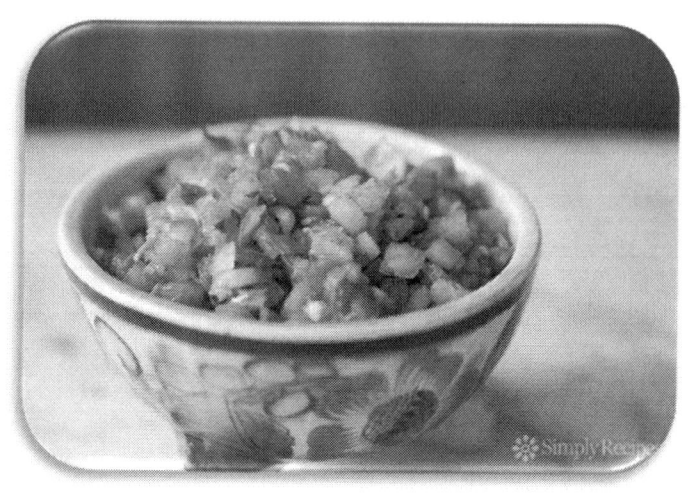

Instruction:

1. Put all ingredients in a bowl, toss well, and serve chilled or at room temperature.

Veggies, Herbs Salad, and Orange-Miso Tahini Dressing

Prep time: 20 minutes

Cooking time: 3 minutes

Servings: 6

Nutrients per serving:

Carbohydrates – 76 g

Fat – 18 g

Protein – 22 g

Calories – 510

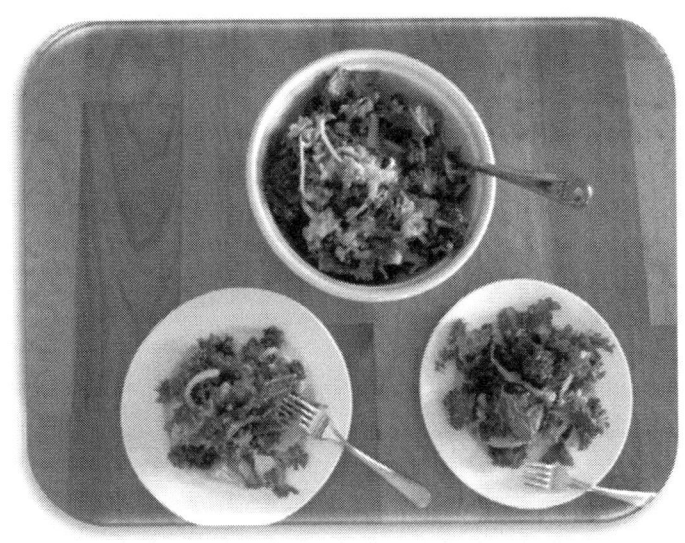

Ingredients:

- 2 small zucchini, sliced into half moons
- 2 cups bite-size broccoli florets
- 1 cup onion, coarsely diced
- 3 cups lightly packed bite-size, hand-torn kale
- 1 cup cherry tomatoes, halved
- ¼ cup pine nuts, lightly toasted
- ¼ cup lightly packed parsley, coarsely chopped
- ¼ cup lightly packed basil, coarsely chopped
- 1 Tbsp garlic, minced
- 1½ cups orange-miso-tahini dressing

Instruction:

1. Fill a saucepan three-quarters full of water, bring to boil, and add zucchini, broccoli, and onion. Blanch 3 minutes until the colors pop vibrantly.
2. Just before draining, mix in torn kale. Remove from heat, strain, and rinse with water until cooled.
3. In a bowl, combine , veggies, pine nuts, herbs, garlic, and half the dressing.
4. Mix in additional dressing until creamy and the consistency you like. Save leftover dressing for later use, to refresh, or to serve on the side.

SOUPS & SALADS

Spicy Squash Soup

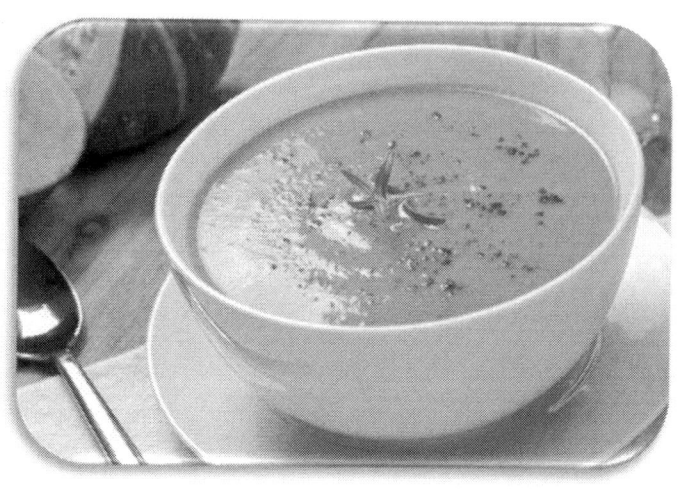

Prep time: 15 minutes

Cooking time: 1 hour 10 minutes

Servings: 6-8

Nutrients per serving:

Carbohydrates – 22 g

Fat – 0 g

Protein – 2 g

Calories – 90

Ingredients:

- 2 carrots, chopped
- 1 butternut squash, cubed
- 1 apple, chopped
- 1 white onion, chopped
- 2 Tbsp ground cinnamon
- 1 tsp ground cumin
- 1 tsp ground chipotle pepper
- Fresh cilantro

Instruction:

1. Preheat oven to 375° F.
2. Mix all ingredients except chipotle and cilantro. Add a ½ cup water, and put it in the oven until the vegetables are soft, around 50 minutes.
3. Combine the vegetables in a pot with five cups of water and the chipotle pepper. Bring to a boil and simmer for 20 minutes.
4. Puree the squash, and serve hot with the cilantro as a garnish.

Spicy Tortilla Soup with Black Beans

Prep time: 15 minutes

Cooking time: 35 minutes

Servings: 8

Nutrients per serving:

Carbohydrates – 27 g

Fat – 4.5 g

Protein – 6 g

Calories – 170

Ingredients:

- 4 corn tortillas
- 1 large yellow onion, peeled and diced
- 1 jalapeño pepper, seeded and diced
- 2 Tbsp Mexican spice blend
- Zest and juice of 1 lime
- 2 28-oz cans no-salt-added diced tomatoes
- ¼ cup chopped fresh cilantro
- 1 15-oz can no-salt-added black beans, drained and rinsed
- 1 avocado, diced

Instruction:

1. Preheat oven to 350°F. Place tortillas on a rimmed baking sheet. Cook tortillas about 10 minutes, flipping halfway through. Remove from oven when chiplike. Break into bite-size pieces.
2. Heat a soup pot over high heat. Add onion, jalapeño, Mexican spice blend, and lime zest. Cook until fragrant and onion starts to soften, about 3 minutes. Add water as needed to avoid burning.
3. Add diced tomatoes and 2 cups water. Bring to a boil, then reduce heat to simmer, and cover. Continue to simmer 15 to 20 minutes. Puree soup with an upright or immersion blender.
4. Add lime juice and cilantro. Serve with baked tortilla chips, black beans, and avocado.

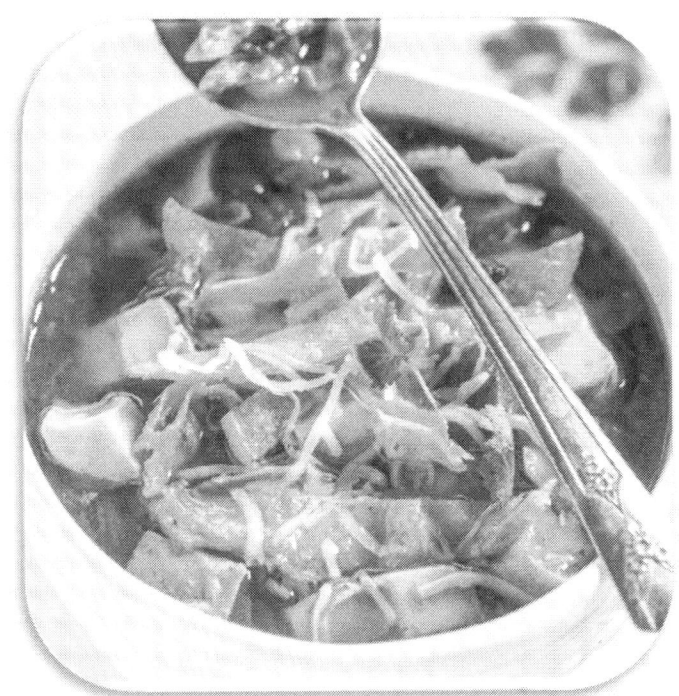

Salmon Chowder

Prep time: 20 minutes

Cooking time: 50 minutes

Servings: 8

Nutrients per serving:

Carbohydrates – 14 g

Fat – 6 g

Protein – 20 g

Calories – 195

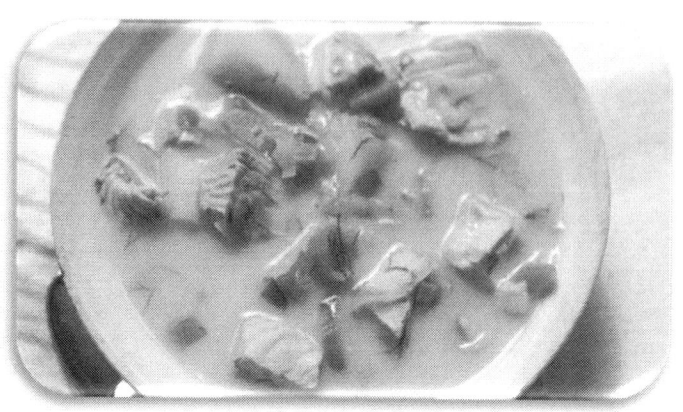

Ingredients:

- 1 onion, chopped
- 1 large shallot, minced
- 2 cloves garlic, minced
- 2 cups peeled, diced red-skin potatoes
- 2 stalks celery, diced
- 2 carrots, diced
- 2 tablespoons olive oil
- 6 cups fish stock
- 1 pound diced tomatoes
- ¼ teaspoon ground cayenne
- 1 tsp Worcestershire sauce
- 1 tsp sherry vinegar
- 1 bay leaf
- 3 Tbsp fresh thyme leaves
- 3 Tbsp chopped Italian parsley
- 3 green onions, diced
- 1 pound cooked salmon, cut into chunks

Instruction:

1. In a large pot, sauté the onion, shallot, garlic, potatoes, celery, and carrots in the olive oil for about 8–12 minutes.
2. Add the stock, tomatoes, cayenne, Worcestershire sauce, and vinegar. Bring to a boil then reduce the heat. Simmer until the potatoes are nearly fork-tender, about 10–20 minutes.
3. Stir in the herbs, green onion, and salmon. Cook until the salmon is heated through, about 5–15 minutes depending on thickness. Discard the bay leaf prior to serving.

Summer Borscht

Prep time: 20 minutes

Cooking time: 1 hour 30 minutes

Servings: 4

Nutrients per serving:

Carbohydrates – 25 g

Fat – 13 g

Protein – 6 g

Calories – 230

Ingredients:

- 8 small beets, peeled
- 1 small onion, chopped
- 1 teaspoon salt
- ½ teaspoon freshly ground pepper
- 4 cups water
- 2 teaspoons sugar
- ¼ cup lemon juice
- 1 egg
- 4 red radishes, diced, for garnish
- 1 cucumber, diced, for garnish

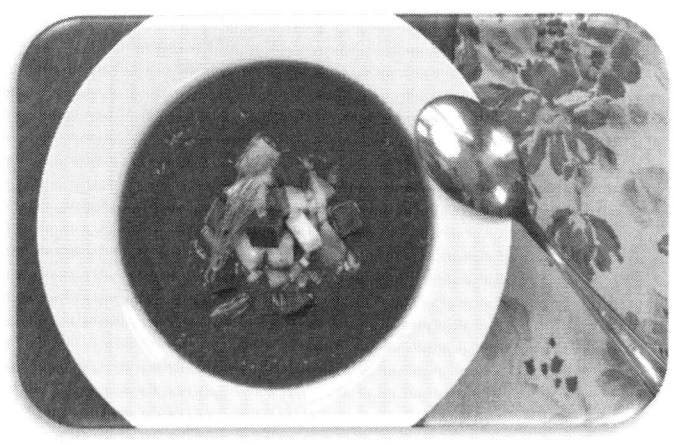

Instruction:

1. In a large pot, bring the beets, onion, salt, pepper, and water to a boil. Boil for 1 hour.
2. Add the sugar and lemon juice and simmer for ½ hour.
3. Remove the beets and grate half. Set aside. Reserve the other half
4. for another recipe. Pour the liquid into a large measuring cup or bowl.
5. In a separate large bowl, beat the egg until very fluffy. Add about ¼ cup of the liquid to the egg and whisk. Continue adding the soup in a slow stream to the egg, whisking continuously.
4. Stir in the grated beets.
6. Chill at least 4 hours or overnight. Ladle into bowls and top with a diced radish, and diced cucumber.

King Oyster Mushroom Soup

Prep time: 20 minutes

Cooking time: 45 minutes

Servings: 4

Nutrients per serving:

Carbohydrates – 25 g

Fat – 9 g

Protein – 21 g

Calories – 377

Ingredients:

- 2 Tbsp olive oil
- 1 onion, minced
- 1 shallot, minced
- 2 carrots, minced
- 2 stalks celery, diced
- 1 bulb fennel, diced
- 6 King Oyster mushrooms, diced
- 4 cups chicken or vegetable stock
- 1 Tbsp thyme leaves
- ½ Tbsp minced rosemary

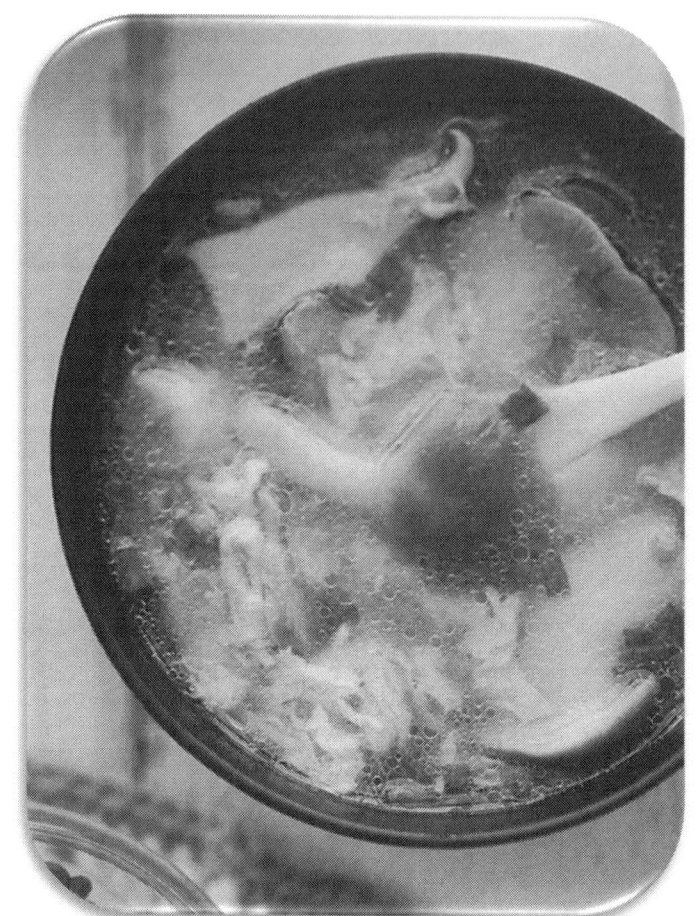

Instruction:

1. Heat the oil in a Dutch oven. Sauté the onion, shallot, carrots, celery, fennel, and mushrooms until soft and fragrant, about 10–15 minutes.
2. Add the stock, thyme, and rosemary. Stir. Cover and simmer 30 minutes

Black Bean Salad with Avocado-Lime Dressing

Prep time: 10 minutes

Cooking time: none

Servings: 4

Nutrients per serving:

Carbohydrates – 49 g

Fat – 17 g

Protein – 19 g

Calories – 400

Ingredients:

- 1 ripe avocado, mashed
- ¼ cup fresh cilantro, chopped
- 2 Tbsp lime juice
- 2 15-oz cans no-salt-added black beans, rinsed and drained
- 4 cups shredded romaine lettuce
- 1 cup grape tomatoes, halved
- 1 cup corn kernels, fresh or thawed if frozen
- 1 small red bell pepper, chopped
- ½ cup toasted pumpkin seeds

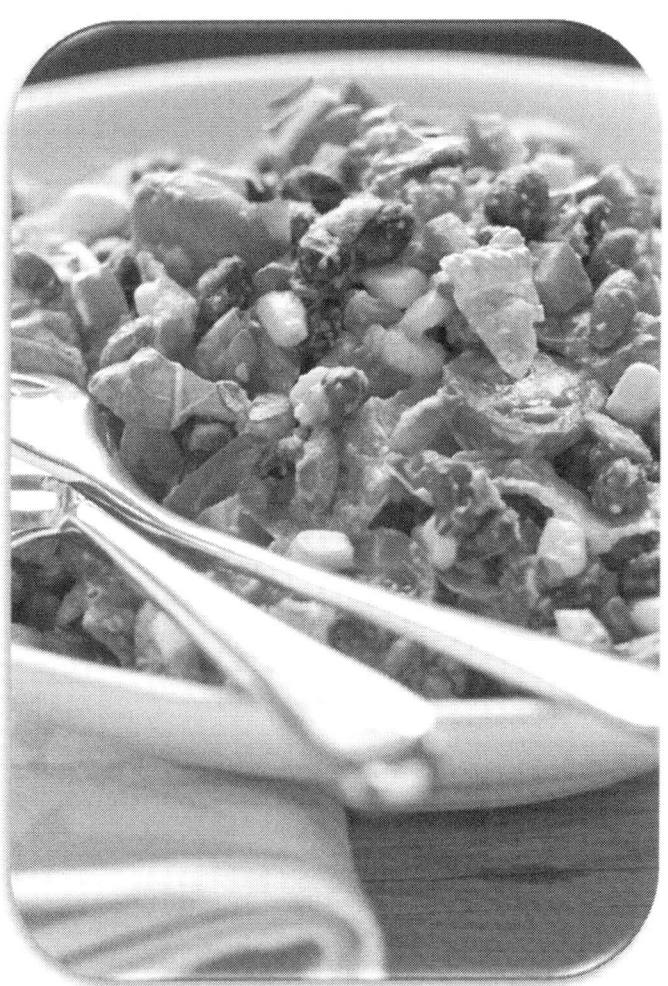

Instruction:

1. In a large bowl, combine all ingredients.

Tangy Bean Salad with Carrots and Green Onions

Prep time: 15 minutes

Cooking time: none

Servings: 4

Nutrients per serving:

Carbohydrates – 23 g

Fat – 4.5 g

Protein – 8 g

Calories – 150

Ingredients:

- 3 Tbsp apple cider vinegar
- 1 Tbsp tamari
- 1 Tsp mustard
- 1 Tbsp sesame tahini
- 3 Tbsp water
- 2 ½ cup garbanzo beans, drained
- ½ cup green onions, thinly sliced
- ½ cup carrots, grated
- ½ bunch parsley, chopped

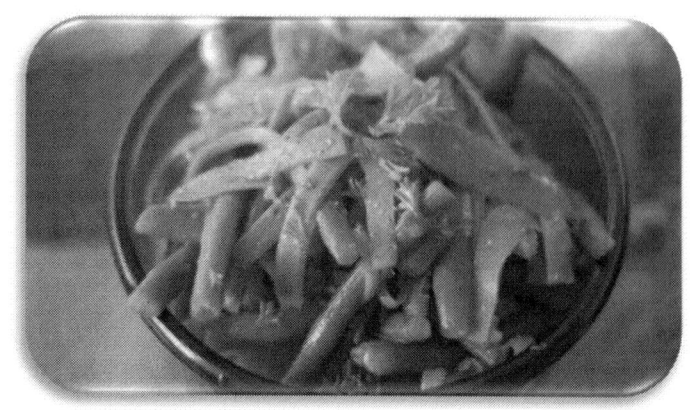

Instruction:

1. Whisk together the vinegar, tamari, mustard, tahini, and water in a bowl.
2. Add remaining ingredients and toss to combine.
3. Set aside for fifteen minutes before serving.

Seafood Salad

Prep time: 15 minutes

Cooking time: none

Servings: 2-3

Nutrients per serving:

Carbohydrates – 2 g

Fat – 10 g

Protein – 18 g

Calories – 180

Ingredients:

- 6 oz cooked fish fillet, diced
- 1 Tsp sweet pickle relish
- ⅛ Tsp dried dill
- Squeeze of lemon juice
- Salt, pepper, to taste
- 4 leaves romaine lettuce, chopped

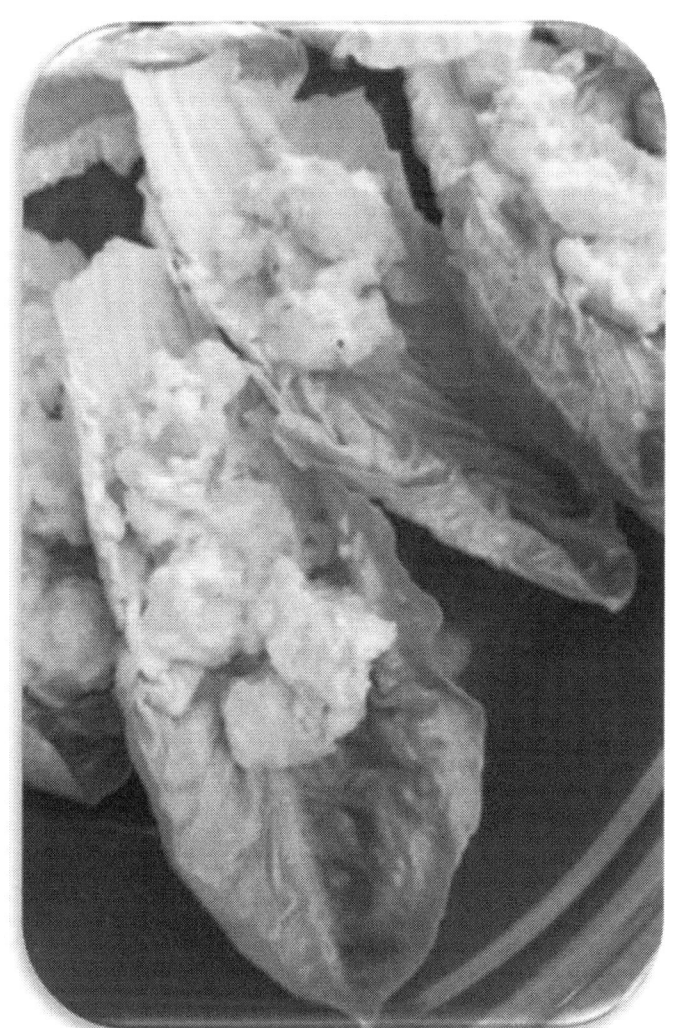

Instruction:

1. Place the fish through the pepper into a bowl and toss it to cCombine all ingredients except lettuce.
2. Arrange the lettuce on a plate, and top with the seafood salad.
3. Chill and serve.

Quinoa, Chard, and Apple Salad

Prep time: 15 minutes

Cooking time: 35 minutes

Servings: 6

Nutrients per serving:

Carbohydrates – 46 g

Fat – 7 g

Protein – 10 g

Calories – 250

Ingredients:

- 2 small shallots, sliced
- 1 bunch chard
- 2 apples, diced
- 2 Tbsp cider vinegar
- ¼ cup sour cherries, dried
- ¼ cup walnuts, toasted

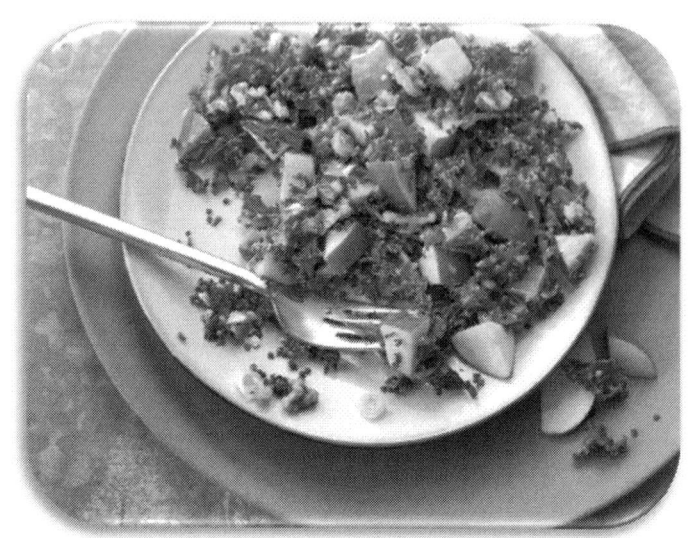

Instruction:

1. Slice the chard and discard the stems. Set it aside.
2. Heat a skillet and add the chard, shallots, and apples. Cook until the shallots have become golden, around 10 minutes. Add the vinegar and scrape up bits from the pan bottom. Add the cherries and another quarter cup of water. Cook another 5 minutes.
3. Top the chard mix with the walnuts.

Salade Niçoise

Prep time: 15 minutes

Cooking time: 30 minutes

Servings: 4

Nutrients per serving:

Carbohydrates – 25 g

Fat – 11 g

Protein – 26 g

Calories – 290

Ingredients:

- ½ lb haricots verts, trimmed
- 1 lb new potatoes
- 6 cup green Leaf Lettuce
- 2 tomatoes, quartered
- 3 hardboiled eggs, quartered
- 4 Anchovy fillets
- 1 jar tuna
- 16 olives
- ⅓ cup prepared Vinaigrette
- Pepper, to taste

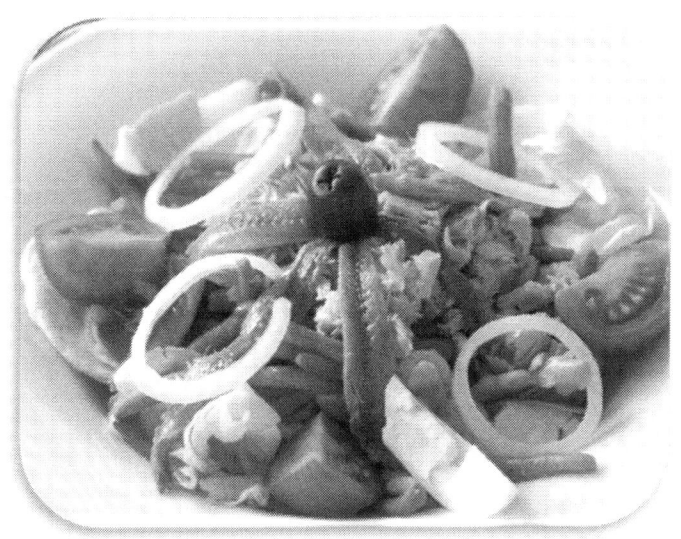

Instruction:

1. Steam the green beans and drain them. Put them into the ice water to cool. Drain and set aside.
2. Cook the potatoes until they're tender, and then run them under cool water. Drain and quarter them.
3. Put the lettuce in the center of a plate, and compose the salad with remaining ingredients. Drizzle with the vinaigrette, and season to taste.

Arugula Salad with Butternut Squash and Prosciutto

Prep time: 15 minutes

Cooking time: 20 minutes

Servings: 6-8

Nutrients per serving:

Carbohydrates – 25 g

Fat – 11 g

Protein – 26 g

Calories – 290

Ingredients:

- 4 cup butter squash, cubed
- 5 Tbsp extra-virgin olive oil, divided
- Salt, pepper, to taste
- 6 cup arugula
- 2 Tbsp lemon juice
- ⅓ lb sliced prosciutto
- ¼ lb ricotta salata, shaved
- ½ cup walnuts, chopped and toasted

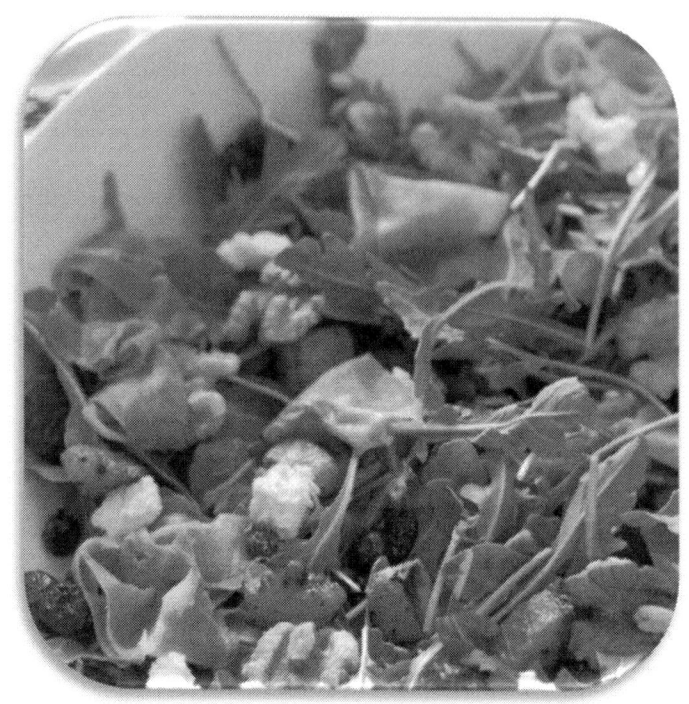

Instruction:

1. Preheat your oven to 375° F.
2. Combine the squash with 3 Tbsp of oil and season with salt and pepper. Toss and then put into a rimmed baking sheet. Roast for 30 minutes, turning every ten minutes. Allow it to cool to room temperature.
3. In a bowl, toss arugula with the rest of the oil and lemon juice. Season with salt and pepper, and arrange on plates. Top with the squash, prosciutto, salata, and walnuts.

BOWLS

Mighty Bowl of Goodness

Prep time: 15 minutes

Cooking time: 20 minutes

Servings: 4

Nutrients per serving:

Carbohydrates – 70 g

Fat – 12 g

Protein – 21 g

Calories – 440

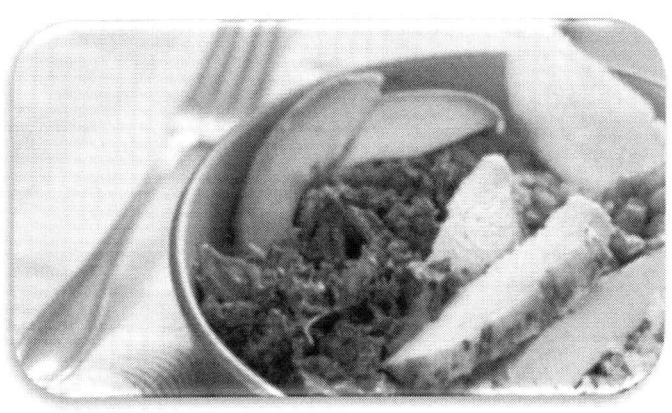

Ingredients:

- 1 cup sprouted green lentils or sprouted mung beans
- 1 bunch kale, stemmed, chopped, and steamed, or 1 head broccoli, cut into florets and steamed
- 16 oz chicken, or salmon
- 1 avocado, cut into wedges
- Parsley, chopped, to taste
- 1 lemon, cut into wedges

Instruction:

1. Cook lentils/mung beans according to package instructions.
2. Divide lentils among four bowls. Top with kale/broccoli, and your choice of chicken or salmon.
3. Garnish with avocado and parsley. Serve with lemon wedges.

Red Pepper Pico

Prep time: 15 minutes

Cooking time: none

Servings: 1

Nutrients per serving:

Carbohydrates – 1 g

Fat – 0 g

Protein – 0 g

Calories – 5

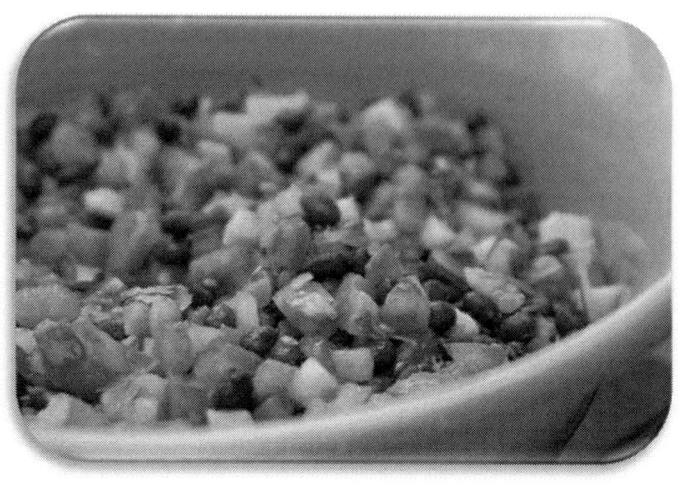

Ingredients:

- ½ cup small-diced red bell pepper
- ¾ cup seeded and small-diced Roma tomato
- ¼ cup small-diced red onion
- ½ jalapeño, seeded and finely minced
- 1 Tbsp lime juice
- 1 clove garlic, finely minced
- 3 Tbsp chopped fresh cilantro
- Sea salt to taste

Instruction:

1. In small mixing bowl, gently toss all ingredients together.

Avocado-Jalapeño Crème

Prep time: 15 minutes

Cooking time: none

Servings: 1

Nutrients per serving:

Carbohydrates – 3 g

Fat – 4 g

Protein – 1 g

Calories – 45

Ingredients:

- 2 avocados
- 2 cloves garlic
- 2 Tbsp lime juice
- 1 jalapeño, seeded
- ¼ cup cilantro, chopped
- ¼ cup unsweetened almond or soy milk
- Sea salt to taste

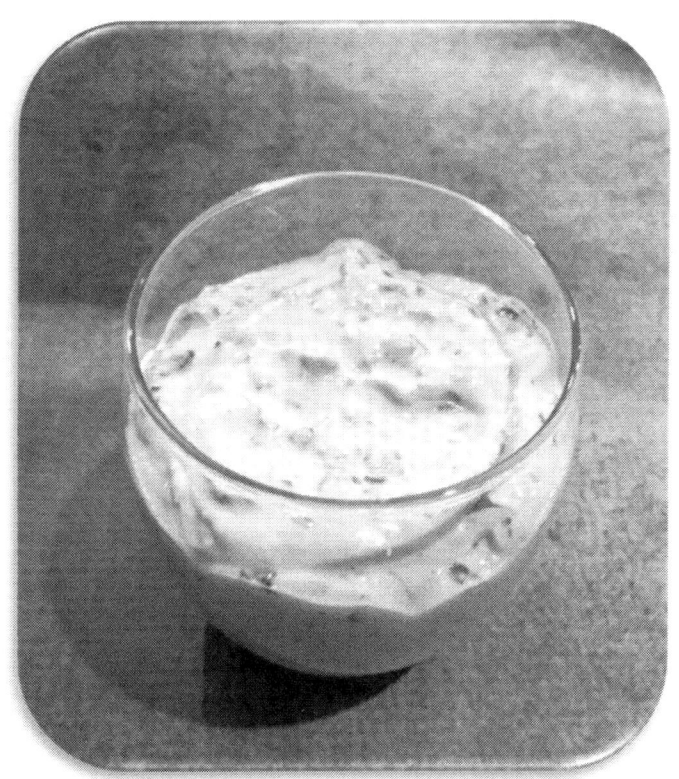

Instruction:

1. In a food processor, mix all ingredients until smooth.

Buddha Bowl

Prep time: 25 minutes

Cooking time: none

Servings: 4

Nutrients per serving:

Carbohydrates – 67 g

Fat – 16 g

Protein – 16 g

Calories – 400

Ingredients:

- 1 cup broccoli florets
- 1 small red onion, chopped
- 1 carrot, grated
- 1 avocado, diced
- ¼ cup sliced Kalamata olives
- 3 ounces extra-firm tofu, cubed
- 1 cooked beet, cubed
- 2 Tbsp rice vinegar
- 1 tsp freshly ground black pepper
- 1 Tbsp avocado oil

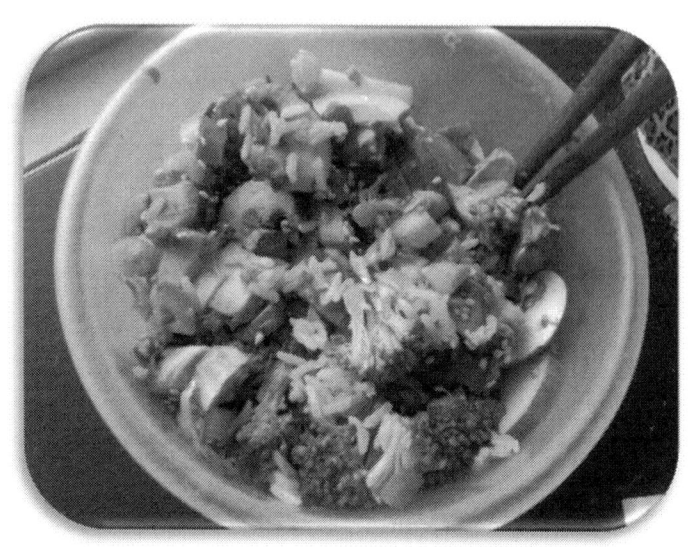

Instruction:

1. Place all ingredients in a large bowl. Toss to combine all ingredients.

DINNER

Mock Chicken Nuggets

Prep time: 25 minutes

Cooking time: none

Servings: 2-3

Nutrients per serving:

Carbohydrates – 3 g

Fat – 9 g

Protein – 22 g

Calories – 180

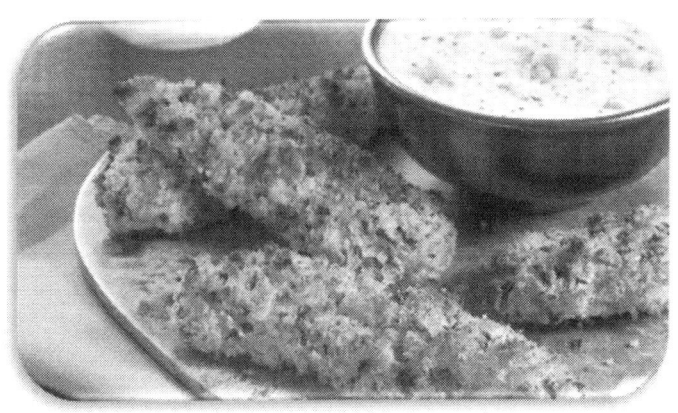

Ingredients:

- ½ lb boneless skinless chicken breasts, cooked, sliced into strips
- 1 Tbsp apple cider vinegar
- 4 Tbsp hot sauce
- ¼ Tsp paprika
- 1 Tsp cane sugar
- ¼ Tsp sea salt
- ⅛ Tsp ground black pepper

Instruction:

1. Combine the vinegar and hot sauce in a bowl. Roll the chicken in the mixture to moisten it.
2. Combine the paprika, sugar, sald, and pepper in a plastic bag, and shake well.
3. Put the chicken strips into the bag and season by shaking it. Serve.

Grilled Chicken and Vegetable Dinner

Prep time: 20 minutes

Cooking time: 30 minutes

Servings: 4

Nutrients per serving:

Carbohydrates – 96 g

Fat – 30 g

Protein – 41 g

Calories – 820

Ingredients:

- 5 Tbsp olive oil
- 2 Tsp granulated garlic
- 2 Tsp onion powder
- Salt, pepper, to taste
- 4 portobello mushroom caps, halved
- 2 yellow squash, halved lengthwise
- 2 zucchini, halved lengthwise
- 4 boneless skinless chicken breasts, halves
- 8 cup baby spinach
- ⅓ cup vinaigrette dressing

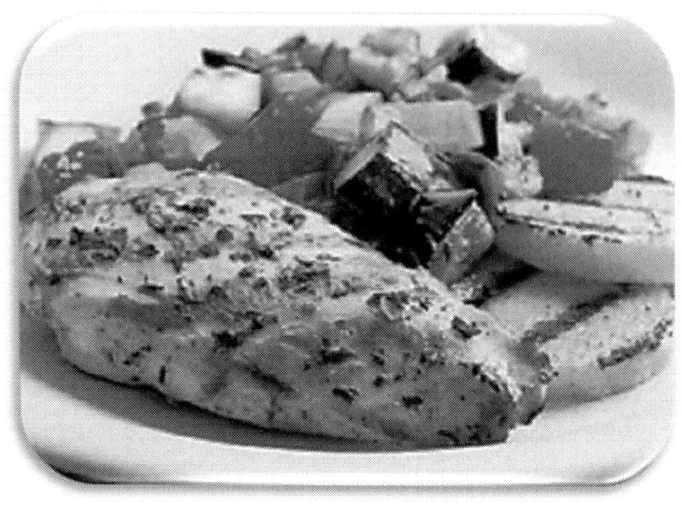

Instruction:

1. In a bowl, add 3 Tbsp oil, 1 tsp garlic, 1 tsp onion powder, salt and pepper to taste. Add the mushrooms, squash, and zucchini, and toss to coat.
2. Marinate the chicken in a shallow dish with the rest of the oil, 1 tsp garlic, 1 tsp onion powder, salt, and pepper to taste.
3. Preheat your grill. Grill the vegetables until they're golden brown, around 10 minutes. Keep them warm on a serving platter.
4. Grill the chicken, flipping once, for around 15-20 minutes.
5. Toss the spinach with the dressing in a bowl, and transfer to plates. Put vegetables and chicken, and serve immediately.

Tarragon Roasted Chicken

Prep time: 20 minutes

Cooking time: 30 minutes

Servings: 4

Nutrients per serving:

Carbohydrates – 96 g

Fat – 30 g

Protein – 41 g

Calories – 820

Ingredients:

- 1 (7-pound) chicken
- 3 tablespoons olive oil
- ½ cup loosely packed tarragon
- 2 Tbsp coarse sea salt
- 1 Tbsp coarsely ground black pepper
- 1 Tbsp Herbes de Provence

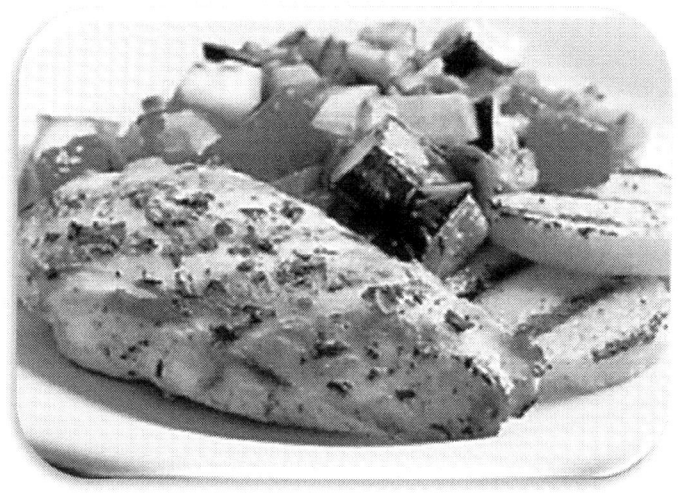

Instruction:

1. In a bowl, add 3 Tbsp oil, 1 tsp garlic, 1 tsp onion powder, salt and pepper to taste. Add the mushrooms, squash, and zucchini, and toss to coat.
2. Marinate the chicken in a shallow dish with the rest of the oil, 1 tsp garlic, 1 tsp onion powder, salt, and pepper to taste.
3. Preheat your grill. Grill the vegetables until they're golden brown, around 10 minutes. Keep them warm on a serving platter.
4. Grill the chicken, flipping once, for around 15-20 minutes.
5. Toss the spinach with the dressing in a bowl, and transfer to plates. Put vegetables and chicken, and serve immediately.

Beef Tacos

Prep time: 20 minutes

Cooking time: 10 minutes

Servings: 4

Nutrients per serving:

Carbohydrates – 136 g

Fat – 24 g

Protein – 46 g

Calories – 940

Ingredients:

- 1 Tbsp canola oil
- 4 6-inch corn tortillas
- 1 lb ground beef
- 2 Tbsp southwest grill seasoning
- 1 cup salsa
  Toppings:
- 1 cup Monterey jack cheese, shredded
- 1 tomato, chopped
- 1 romaine lettuce heart, sliced
- 1 red onion, chopped
- ½ cup plain, whole milk yogurt

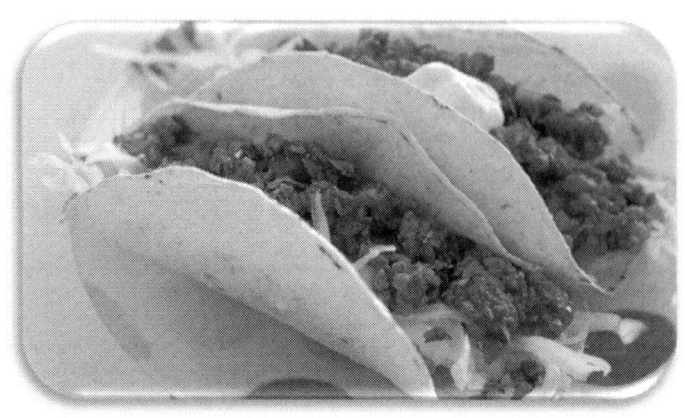

Instruction:

1. Warm the oil in skill over medium heat and add the beef and seasoning. Cook for about 5 minutes.
2. Stir in ½ cup of salsa, and lower the heat to allow it to simmer another 5 minutes.
3. Spoon the beef on tortillas.
4. Put the rest of the salsa into bowls, and serve to allow everyone to make their own tacos.

Mini Turkey Meatloaf and Green Beans Dinner

Prep time: 20 minutes

Cooking time: 45 minutes

Servings: 4

Nutrients per serving:

Carbohydrates – 24 g

Fat – 11 g

Protein – 25 g

Calories – 290

Ingredients:

- 2 tsp extra-virgin olive oil
- 1 lb ground Turkey breast
- ½ cup yellow onion, minced
- 1 cup sweet potato, grated
- ¼ cup prepared barbecue sauce, divided
- 1 ¾ tsp sea salt, divided
- ½ tsp black pepper, divided
- 1 lb green beans, trimmed

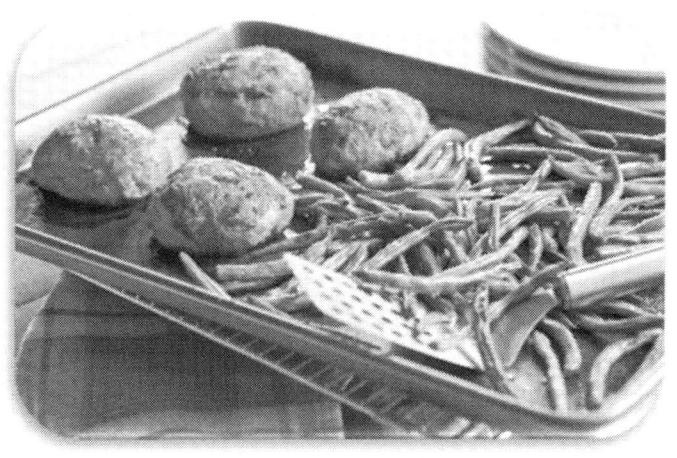

Instruction:

1. Preheat oven to 400° F and oil a large sheet tray.
2. Mix the turkey, onion, and sweet potato together with 3 Tbsp of the barbecue sauce, 1 tsp salt, and 1/4 tsp pepper. Form into four loaves and brush with the rest of the barbecue sauce. Bake for 20 minutes.
3. Toss the green beans with oil, and the rest of the salt and pepper. Arrange these on the pan with the meatloaves and roast until the green beans are tender, about 25 more minutes.

Bacon-Wrapped Stuffed Sea Scallops

Prep time: 20 minutes

Cooking time: 10 minutes

Servings: 12

Nutrients per serving:

Carbohydrates – 24 g

Fat – 11 g

Protein – 25 g

Calories – 290

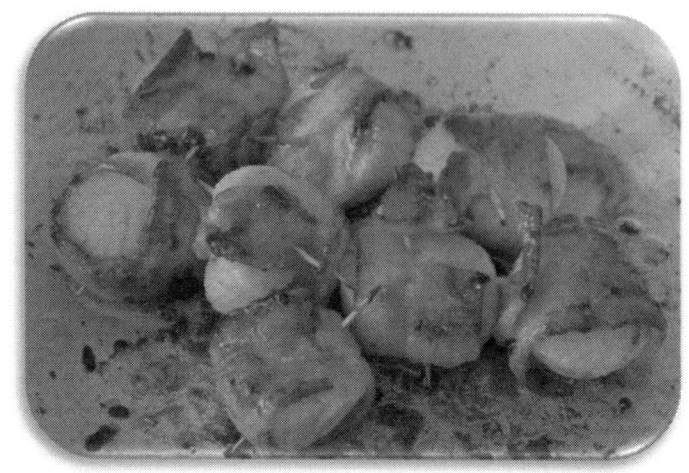

Ingredients:

- 12 slices bacon
- 1 lb sea scallops
- 3 oz blue cheese
- ¼ cup fig spread
- Pepper, to taste
- Canola spray oil

Instruction:

1. Coat a baking sheet with oil.
2. Slice scallops in half horizontally, leaving one side attached. Put a sliver of blue cheese in the middle, add a dab of fig spread, and close. Wrap with a slice of bacon and secure with a toothpick. Season with pepper.
3. Preheat your broiler to 350°.
4. Broil for 4-5 minutes on each side until the bacon is done. Remove the toothpicks, and serve with extra fig spread.

Grilled Chicken and Peppers over Arugula

Prep time: 20 minutes

Cooking time: 6-7 minutes

Servings: 4

Nutrients per serving:

Carbohydrates – 5 g

Fat – 11 g

Protein – 32 g

Calories – 250

Ingredients:

- 2 skinless, boneless chicken breast halves
- 7 Tbsp Italian dressing, divided
- 2 bell peppers, quartered
- ¼ onion, sliced
- 6 cup arugula leaves

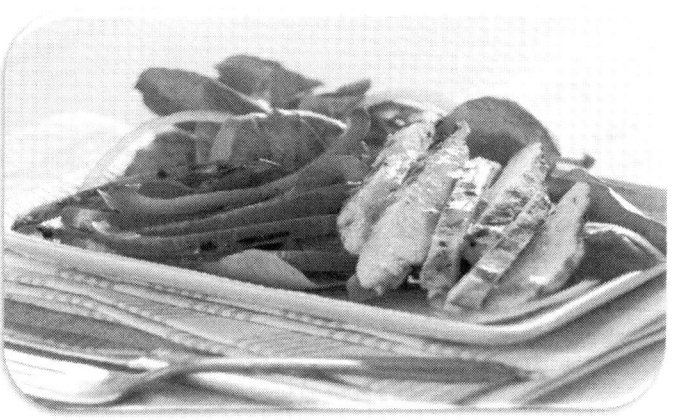

Instruction:

1. Halve the chicken breasts.
2. Prepare a grill to medium-high heat and brush the chicken with 3 Tbsp dressing on either side.
3. In a bowl, toss the peppers with 2 Tbsp of dressing.
4. Grill the chicken and peppers, turning them until the chicken is cooked through and the peppers have become tender, about take 6-7 minutes.
5. Toss the onion and arugula with the rest of the dressing, and arrange it on a platter. Slice the chicken and peppers, and put them on top of the arugula.

Grilled Caribbean Pork Tenderloin

Prep time: 20 minutes

Cooking time: 25 minutes

Servings: 6

Nutrients per serving:

Carbohydrates – 33 g

Fat – 6 g

Protein – 33 g

Calories – 310

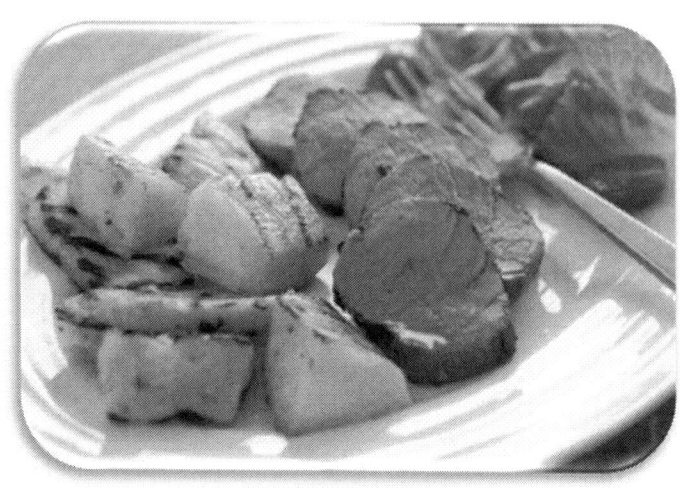

Ingredients:

- 1 cup orange juice
- ½ cup green onions, thinly sliced
- ¼ cup distilled white vinegar
- ¼ cup tamari
- 3 Tbsp lime juice
- 1 serrano pepper, stemmed, seeded and minced
- 2 tsp allspice, ground
- ¾ tsp cinnamon, ground
- ¾ tsp nutmeg, ground
- 1 clove garlic, minced
- 2 pork tenderloins
- Canola oil
- 1 pineapple, diced
- 2 plantains, peeled, sliced

Instruction:

1. Combine all ingredients except last three. Cover and chill for 4 hours.
2. Oil the grill and preheat it to medium heat. Drain the pork and get rid of the marinade. Grill the pork for about 15 minutes, or until done.
3. Brush the pineapple and plantains with some oil and grill them, flipping once, around 5-8 minutes.
4. Cut the pork into medallions. Serve with the pineapple and plantains on the side.

Roasted Lemon-Herb Chicken

Prep time: 20 minutes (+14 hours)

Cooking time: 1 hour

Servings: 8

Nutrients per serving:

Carbohydrates – 18 g

Fat – 4 g

Protein – 24 g

Calories – 124

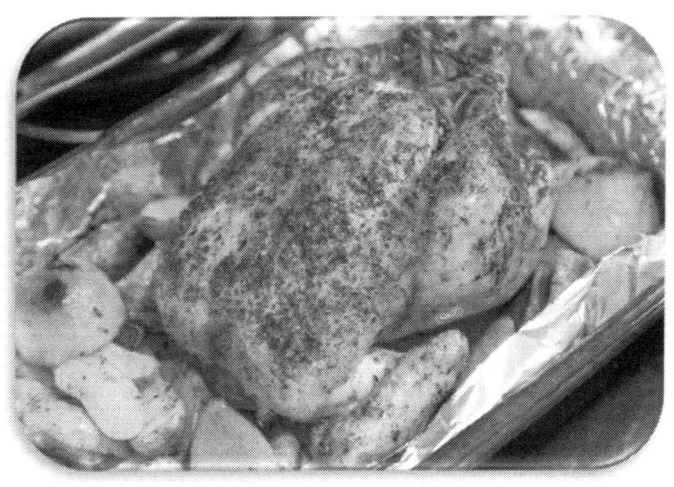

Ingredients:

- 1 Tbsp plus 1 ½ tsp lemon juice
- 2 Tbsp salt
- 2 qt. water
- 1 ½ lb bone-in chicken
- 1 ¾ tsp extra-virgin olive oil
- 2 Tbsp fresh oregano, chopped
- 2 Tbsp Italian flat-leaf parsley, chopped
- 2 Tbsp fresh basil, sliced
- ⅛ tsp pepper

Instruction:

1. The evening before, combine the lemon juice and salt with two quarts of water in a bowl. Add the chicken and cover. Refrigerate overnight.
2. Remove the chicken, and pat it dry the following day. In a bowl, combine the oil and herbs. Add the chicken, and coat it well. Cover and refrigerate another 6 hours.
3. Preheat your oven to 350° F and bake 1 hour.

Pesto Chicken Breasts

Prep time: 20 minutes

Cooking time: 20 minutes

Servings: 4

Nutrients per serving:

Carbohydrates – 4 g

Fat – 29 g

Protein – 54 g

Calories – 498

Ingredients:

- 3 cups basil, loosely packed
- ¼ cup olive oil
- ¼ cup finely grated Parmesan cheese
- ¼ cup pine nuts
- 1 teaspoon kosher salt
- 1 teaspoon freshly ground black pepper
- 4 boneless, skinless chicken breasts

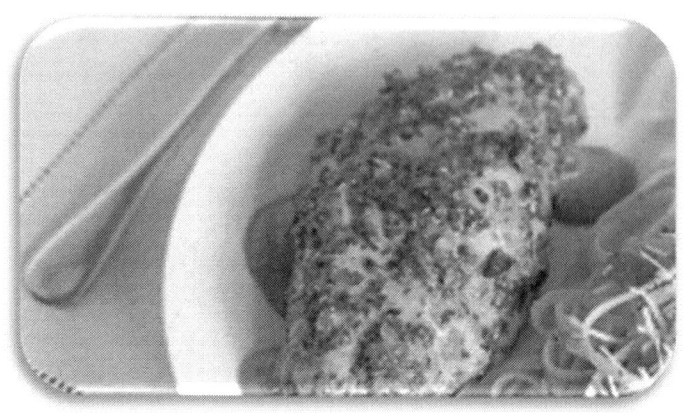

Instruction:

1. Preheat oven to 350°F.
2. Place the basil, olive oil, Parmesan, pine nuts, salt, and pepper in a food processor. Pulse until a thick paste forms.
3. Line a baking sheet with foil. Rub both sides of each chicken breast with the pesto and place on baking sheet. Bake until the chicken is fully cooked, about 20 minutes.

Lemon-Thyme Roasted Capon

Prep time: 20 minutes

Cooking time: 2 hours 20 minutes

Servings: 8

Nutrients per serving:

Carbohydrates – 4 g

Fat – 80 g

Protein – 85 g

Calories – 956

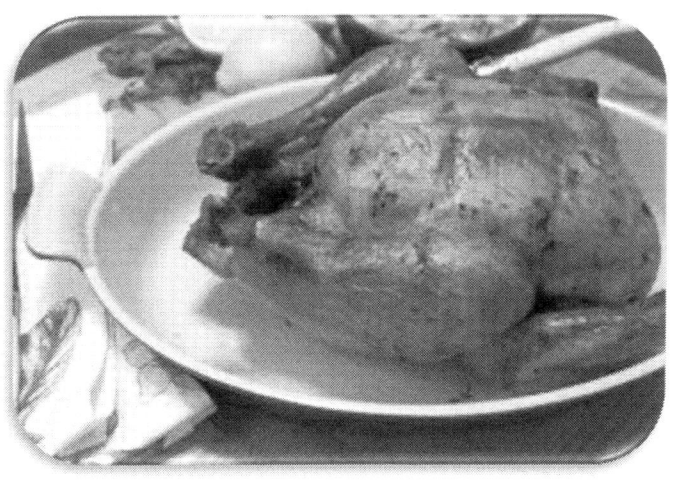

Ingredients:

- 1 (8-pound) capon
- 1 lemon, halved
- 1 small onion, quartered
- 4 cloves garlic
- 2 Tbsp olive oil
- 3 Tbsp kosher salt
- 1 Tbsp coarsely ground black pepper
- 1½ Tbsp chervil
- 1½ Tbsp marjoram
- 1½ Tbsp thyme leaves

Instruction:

1. Preheat oven to 450°F.
2. Place the capon on a roasting rack. Place the lemon, onion, and garlic in the cavity.
3. Rub the capon with olive oil then sprinkle with salt, pepper, chervil, marjoram, and thyme.
4. Roast for 2 hours then reduce heat to 350°F and cook an additional 20 minutes or until fully cooked.

Mustard Grilled Lamb Chops

Prep time: 20 minutes

Cooking time: 20 minutes

Servings: 4

Nutrients per serving:

Carbohydrates – 8 g

Fat – 49 g

Protein – 19 g

Calories – 546

Ingredients:

- 4 lamb loin chops
- 1 lemon, sliced thinly
- 1 shallot, minced
- 4 cloves garlic, minced
- 2 Tbsp minced rosemary
- ¼ cup red wine vinegar
- ¼ cup olive oil
- ¼ cup Dijon mustard
- ½ tsp sea salt

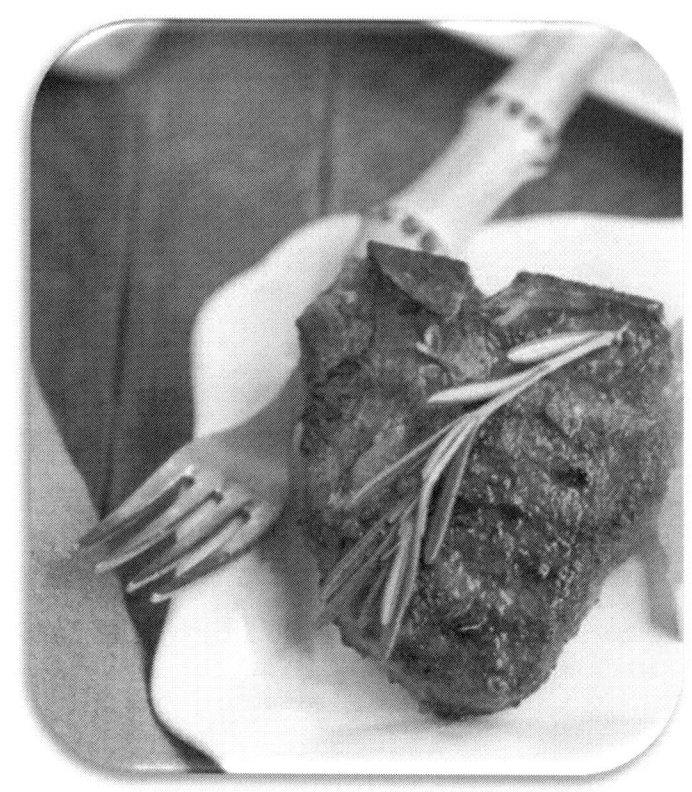

Instruction:

1. Place all ingredients in a marinating container or resealable plastic bag. Refrigerate for 4 hours.
2. Prepare your grill according to manufacturer's instructions. Place the lamb chops on the grill and cook, turning once, until mediumrare, just a few minutes on each side.

Herb-Rubbed Bison Steaks

Prep time: 20 minutes

Cooking time: 20 minutes

Servings: 2

Nutrients per serving:

Carbohydrates – 1 g

Fat – 13 g

Protein – 35 g

Calories – 261

Ingredients:

- 1 tsp ground rosemary
- 1 tsp dried parsley
- 1 tsp dried oregano
- 1 tsp dried basil
- ½ tsp paprika
- ½ tsp ground mustard
- ½ tsp sea salt
- 2 (6-ounce) bison steaks
- 1½ Tbsp olive oil

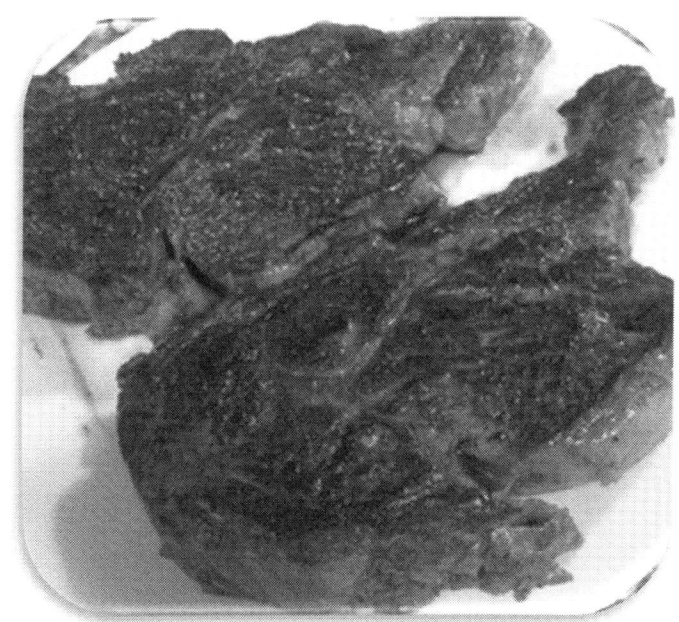

Instruction:

1. In a small bowl, mix together the spices. Rub them into all sides of the bison steaks.
2. Heat the oil in a nonstick skillet. Pan-fry the bison, flipping once, until desired doneness.

Pear-Sage Meatloaf

Prep time: 20 minutes

Cooking time: 40 minutes

Servings: 2

Nutrients per serving:

Carbohydrates – 12 g

Fat – 1 g

Protein – 3 g

Calories – 71

Ingredients:

- 1 pound 94% lean ground beef
- 1 egg, beaten
- 2 shallots, grated
- ¾ cup fresh bread crumbs
- 1 cup shredded Bosc pear
- 2 Tbsp grainy mustard
- 1½ Tbsp minced sage
- 1 tsp freshly ground black pepper
- 1 tsp sea salt
- 1 tsp smoked paprika
- ¼ tsp allspice

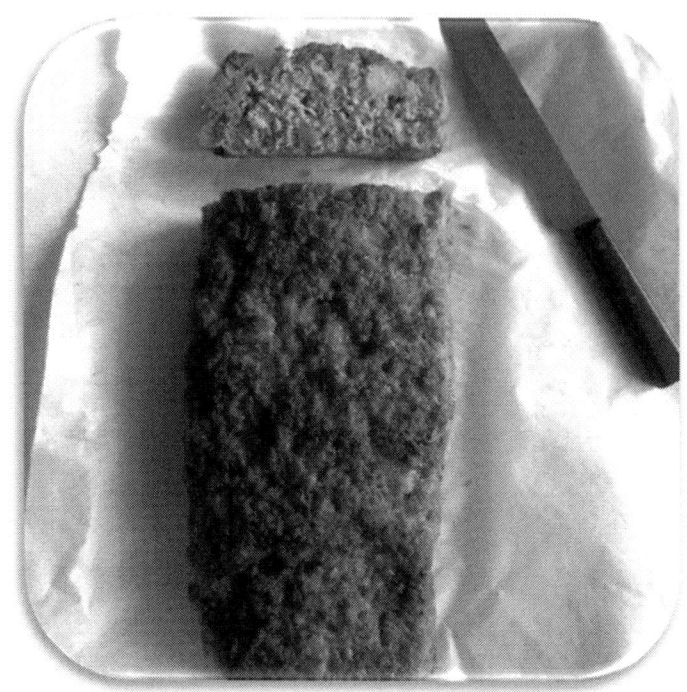

Instruction:

1. Preheat oven to 350°F.
2. Place all ingredients in a medium bowl. Mix together until all ingredients are evenly distributed.
3. Mold into a loaf and place in a loaf pan. Bake for 40 minutes or until fully cooked. Allow to sit for 5 minutes before serving.

Venison Burgers

Prep time: 20 minutes

Cooking time: 5-8 minutes

Servings: 4

Nutrients per serving:

Carbohydrates – 7 g

Fat – 6 g

Protein – 27 g

Calories – 196

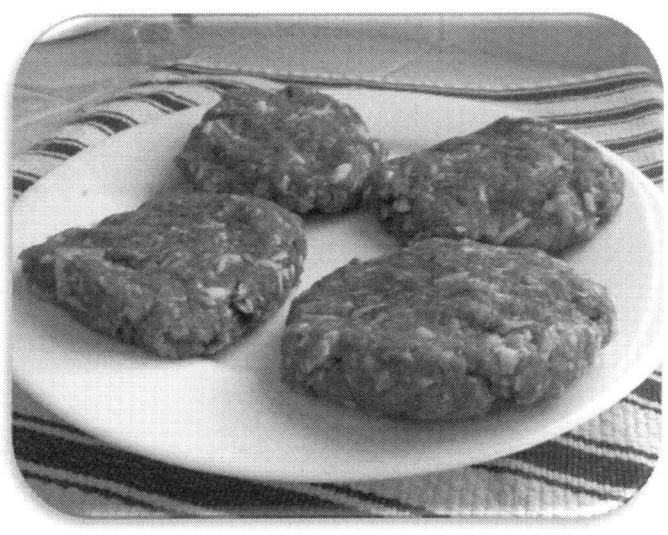

Ingredients:

- 1 pound ground venison
- 1 Tbsp tomato paste
- 1 tsp minced fresh basil
- 1 tsp freshly ground black pepper
- ½ tsp ground cayenne
- 1½ Tbsp Worcestershire sauce
- 1 shallot, minced
- 1 clove garlic, minced
- 1 Tbsp canola oil

Instruction:

1. In a small bowl, mix together the venison, tomato paste, basil, pepper, cayenne, Worcestershire sauce, shallot, and garlic until well blended. Form into 4 patties.
2. Heat the oil in a skillet. Add the burgers and cook, turning once, until desired doneness is achieved and the burgers are browned on both sides, about 5–8 minutes.

DESSERTS

Sweet Potato Chocolate Mousse

Prep time: 20 minutes

Cooking time: none

Servings: 2

Nutrients per serving:

Carbohydrates – 49 g

Fat – 6 g

Protein – 6 g

Calories – 250

Ingredients:

- ¾ cup pitted dates, soaked in warm water 10 minutes to soften
- 2 cups sweet potato purée
- 2 Tbsp no-salt-added unsweetened almond butter
- ¾ cup unsweetened almond milk
- ½ cup unsweetened cocoa powder
- ½ tsp ground cinnamon
- 1 tsp pure vanilla extract
- 3 Tbsp flaxseed meal

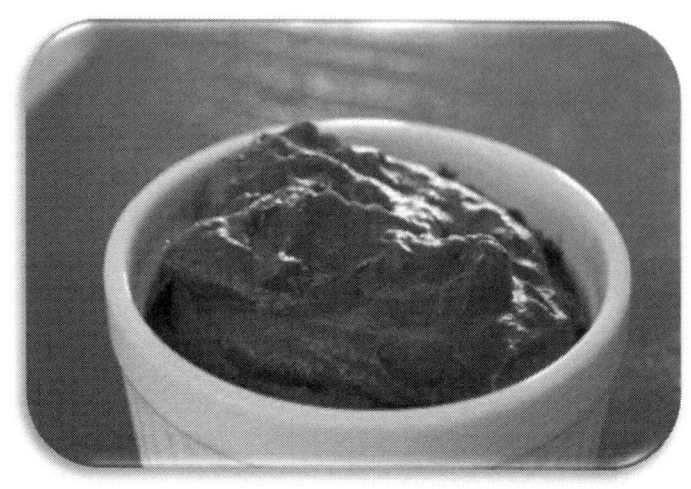

Instruction:

1. Drain soaking liquid from dates, squeeze out any excess water, and place dates in a food processor or high-speed blender. Add sweet potato, almond butter, almond milk, cocoa, cinnamon, vanilla, and flaxseed meal, and puree until well combined and creamy.
2. Refrigerate mousse in an airtight container up to 3 days or freeze up to 5 days.
3. If using for a pie filling, pour mousse into a baked piecrust. Refrigerate for about 2 hours before serving.

Raspberry Nice Cream

Prep time: 15 minutes (+4 hours)

Cooking time: none

Servings: 4

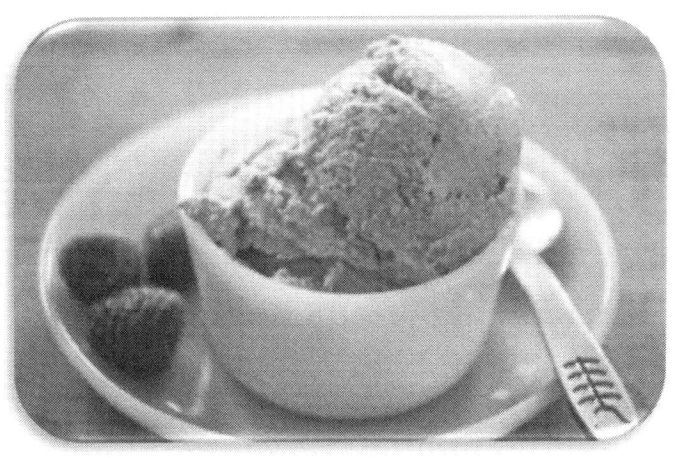

Nutrients per serving:

Carbohydrates – 26 g

Fat – 8 g

Protein – 4 g

Calories – 170

Ingredients:

- 6 oz raspberries, thawed
- ½ cup raw whole cashews, soaked in warm water at room temperature at least 2 hours, drained
- 2 bananas, thickly sliced and frozen

Instruction:

1. Puree raspberries and cashews in a blender or food processor until smooth, adding up to ¼ cup water if needed.
2. Add bananas and puree again, scraping down the sides often.
3. Transfer to a sealed freezer-safe container and freeze until just solid, about 4 hours.

Coconut Cookies

Prep time: 20 minutes

Cooking time: 30 minutes

Servings: 12

Nutrients per serving:

Carbohydrates – 26 g

Fat – 8 g

Protein – 4 g

Calories – 170

Ingredients:

- ½ cup banana, mashed
- ¼ cup coconut oil, melted
- 1 cup quick-cooking rolled oats
- ⅓ cup coconut, shredded
- ⅓ cup walnuts, minced
- 2 Tbsp protein powder
- 1 Tbsp chia seeds
- Pinch fine sea salt

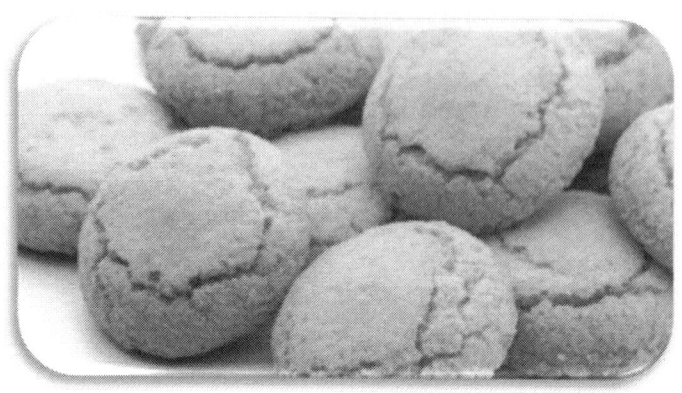

Instruction:

1. Preheat oven to 325°F. Line a baking sheet with some parchment paper.
2. In a bowl, stir the banana and coconut oil together until smooth. Stir in remaining ingredients.
3. Using your hands, roll the mix into 12 balls about the size of a golf ball. Place them on the baking sheet.
4. Flatten the cookies until they're about 2 inches in diameter.
5. Bake for about 25 minutes. Let them cool for a few minutes. Serve.

Fruit and Waffle Kabobs

Prep time: 15 minutes

Cooking time: 25 minutes

Servings: 4

Nutrients per serving:

Carbohydrates – 57 g

Fat – 14 g

Protein – 2 g

Calories – 400

Ingredients:

- Canola Spray oil
- 4 peaches, diced
- 8 slices bacon
- 16 mini waffles, thawed

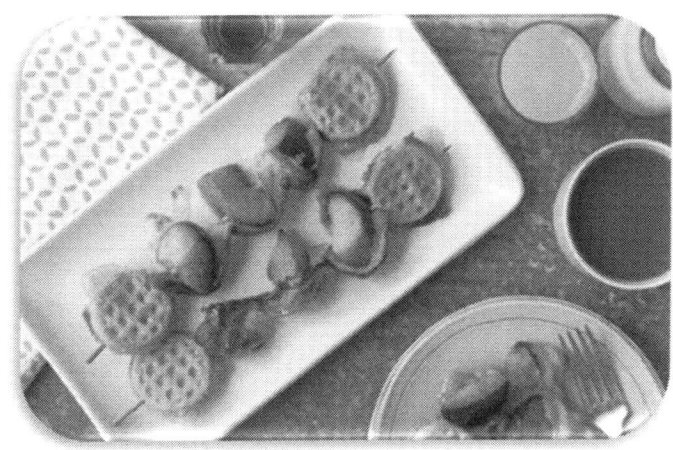

Instruction:

1. Preheat oven to 400° F. Line a baking sheet with foil, and put a large wire rack in the center. Coat the rack with cooking spray.
2. Toss the fruit with the syrup.
3. Thread the bacon and fruit onto 8-inch wooden skewers.
4. Adjust the ingredients to leave 2 inches of empty space at the ends of the skewers. Put the kabobs on the rack.
5. Bake 15 minutes.
6. Remove from the oven and flip the skewers. Thread mini waffle onto either end . and cook 10 minutes.

Oatmeal-Raisin Cookies

Prep time: 35 minutes

Cooking time: 12 minutes

Servings: 7

Nutrients per serving:

Carbohydrates – 9 g

Fat – 3 g

Protein – 2 g

Calories – 70

Ingredients:

- 1 cup raisins
- 1 cup gluten-free rolled oats
- 1 tsp baking powder
- 1 tsp ground cinnamon
- ¼ tsp ground nutmeg
- ¼ tsp fine sea salt
- ½ cup no-salt-added cashew butter
- 1 tsp pure vanilla extract

Instruction:

1. Preheat oven to 350°F. Line 2 baking sheets with parchment paper. Soak ½ cup of the raisins in warm water at least 10 minutes, leaving the remaining ½ cup dry. Drain and reserve ¼ cup of the soaking liquid.
2. Pulse ¾ cup of the oats in a blender or food processor until finely ground and powdery, setting aside the remaining ¼ cup. (Do not wash the food processor.) In a large bowl, whisk together oat flour, baking powder, cinnamon, nutmeg and salt; set aside.

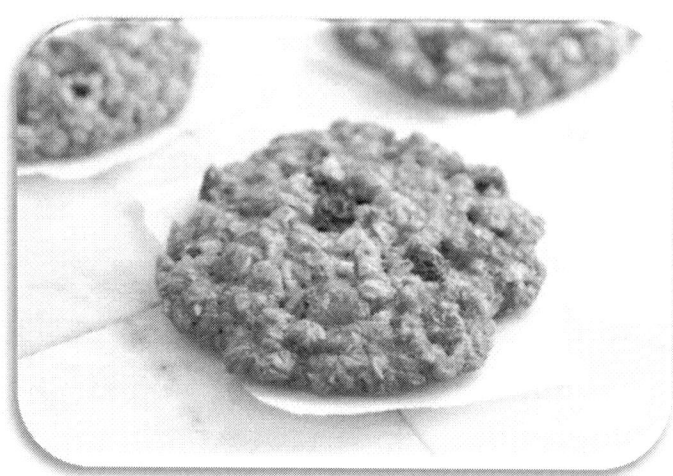

3. Combine raisins and ¼ cup of the soaking liquid in the food processor. Pulse to chop, then puree until smooth. Add cashew butter and vanilla, then puree until creamy.
4. Add raisin mixture, remaining ½ cup whole raisins, and remaining ¼ cup oats to oat mixture. Stir thoroughly until all the oat flour is absorbed.
5. Drop heaping teaspoons of dough on the prepared baking sheets, spacing cookies about 1 inch apart.
6. Gently flatten each with the back of a spoon. Bake until cookies are lightly browned on the bottom, 10 to 12 minutes.
7. Let cookies cool on the baking sheet for 5 minutes, then transfer them to a wire ack and let cool completely. Cookies will keep in an airtight container at room temperature up to 3 days or in the freezer up to 2 weeks. Serve.

Star Anise Pears

Prep time: 10 minutes

Cooking time: 15 minutes

Servings: 4

Nutrients per serving:

Carbohydrates – 42 g

Fat – 0 g

Protein – 1 g

Calories – 161

Ingredients:

- 4 pears, halved lengthwise
- 1 tsp ground star anise
- ½ cup water

Instructions:

1. Use a small spoon to scoop out the seeds of each pear. Heat a large nonstick skillet over medium heat.
2. In a small bowl, whisk together the star anise and sugar. Pour onto a plate.
3. Press the cut side of each pear into the sugar.
4. Place the pear halves, sugar side down, into the skillet and cook 5–8 minutes or until the pears begin to brown. Add the water. Cover and simmer for another 5 minutes or until the pears are tender.
5. Remove the pears to a platter. Reduce the water-sugar mixture remaining in the skillet until syrupy, about 2 minutes, and pour over pears. Serve.

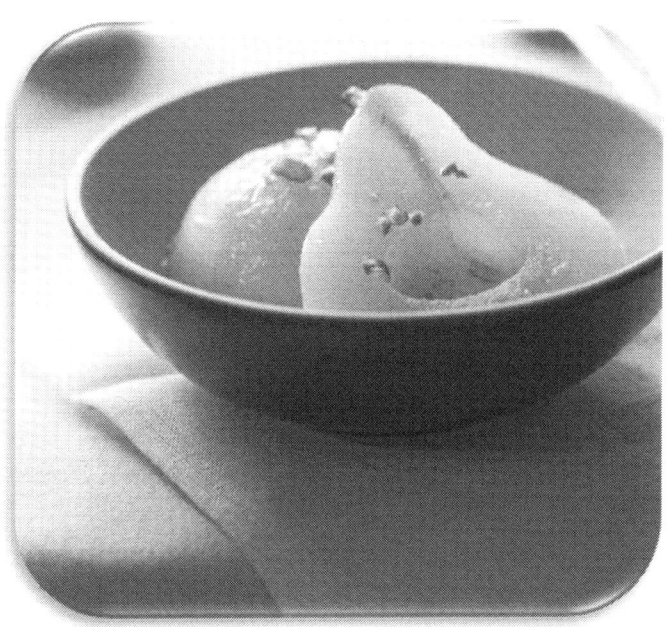

CONCLUSION

Thank you for reading this book and having the patience to try the recipes.

I do hope that you gain as much enjoyment reading and experimenting with the meals as I have had writing this book.

If you would like to leave a comment, you can do it at the Order section->Digital orders, in your amazon account.

Stay safe and healthy!

Recipe Index

A

Amaranth Banana Breakfast Porridge 29
Arugula Salad with Butternut Squash and Prosciutto 46
Avocado-Jalapeño Crème 49

B

Bacon-Wrapped Stuffed Sea Scallops 56
Beef Tacos 54
Black Bean Salad with Avocado-Lime Dressing 41
Breakfast Banana Splits 24
Breakfast Green Machine Smoothie 21
Breakfast Sandwich 22
Breakfast Turkey Sausage 27
Buddha Bowl 50

C

Coconut Cookies 68

D

Deviled Ham Tea Sandwiches 31

F

Fresh Salsa 34
Fruit and Waffle Kabobs 69

G

Grilled Caribbean Pork Tenderloin 58
Grilled Chicken and Peppers over Arugula 57
Grilled Chicken and Vegetable Dinner 52

H

Herb-Rubbed Bison Steaks 63

K

Kasha Breakfast Porridge 26
King Oyster Mushroom Soup 40

L

Lemon-Thyme Roasted Capon 61

M

Mighty Bowl of Goodness 47
Mini Sausage Breakfast Sandwiches 28
Mini Turkey Meatloaf and Green Beans Dinner 55
Mock Chicken Nuggets 51
Mustard Grilled Lamb Chops 62

O

Oatmeal Fruit Shake 19
Oatmeal-Raisin Cookies 70
Oil-Free Herb Pesto 32
Orangeade 30

P

Pear-Sage Meatloaf 64
Pesto Chicken Breasts 60
Pumpkin Pie Smoothie 20

Q

Quinoa, Chard, and Apple Salad 44

R

Raspberry Nice Cream 67
Red Pepper Pico 48
Refried Bean and Avocado Soft Tacos 33
Roasted Lemon-Herb Chicken 59

S

Salade Niçoise 45
Salmon Chowder 38
Seafood Salad 43
Spicy Squash Soup 36
Spicy Tortilla Soup with Black Beans 37
Star Anise Pears 71
Summer Borscht 39
Sweet Potato Chocolate Mousse 66

T

Tangy Bean Salad with Carrots and Green Onions 42
Tarragon Roasted Chicken 53

V

Veggies, Herbs Salad, and Orange-Miso Tahini Dressing 35
Venison Burgers 65

W

Whole Wheat Blueberry Pancakes 25

Conversion Tables

VALUME EQUIVALENTS (LIQUID)

US STANDARD	US STANDARD (OUNCES)	METRIC (VOLUME)
2 tablespoons	1 fl. oz.	30 mL
¼ cup	2 fl. oz.	60 mL
½ cup	4 fl. oz.	120 mL
1 cup	8 fl. oz.	240 mL
1 ½ cup	12 fl. oz.	355 mL
2 cups or 1 pint	16 fl. oz.	475 mL
4 cups or 1 quart	32 fl. oz.	1 L
1 gallon	128 fl. oz.	4 L

OVEN TEMPERATURES

FAHRENHEIT(F)	CELSIUS(C) APPROXIMATE
250 °F	120 °C
300 °F	150 °C
325 °F	165 °C
350 °F	180 °C
375 °F	190 °C
400 °F	200 °C
425 °F	220 °C
450 °F	230 °C

VALUME EQUIVALENTS (LIQUID)

US STANDARD	METRIC (APPROXIMATE)
⅛ teaspoon	0.5 mL
¼ teaspoon	1 mL
½ teaspoon	2 mL
⅔ teaspoon	4 mL
1 teaspoon	5 mL
1 tablespoon	15 mL
¼ cup	59 mL
⅓ cup	79 mL
½ cup	118 mL
⅔ cup	156 mL
¾ cup	177 mL
1 cup	235 mL
2 cups or 1 pint	475 mL
3 cups	700 mL
4 cups or 1 quart	1 L
½ gallon	2 L
1 gallon	4 L

WEIGHT EQUIVALENTS

US STANDARD	METRIC (APPROXIMATE)
½ ounce	15 g
1 ounces	30 g
2 ounces	60 g
4 ounces	115 g
8 ounces	225 g
12 ounces	340 g
16 ounce or 1 pound	455 g

Other Books by Emma Green

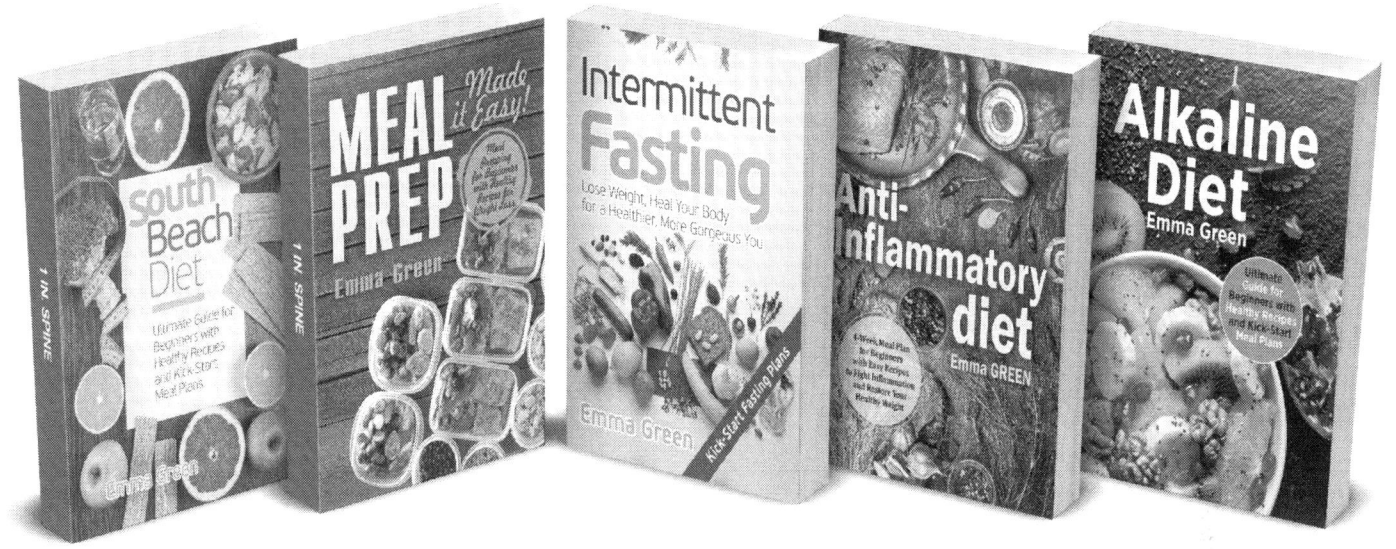

Emma Green's page on Amazon

https://goo.gl/7yn2fR

Made in the USA
Columbia, SC
24 August 2019